Instructor's Curriculum Resource to accompany

Medical Terminology

A SHORT COURSE

FOURTH EDITION

Davi-Ellen Chabner, BA, MAT

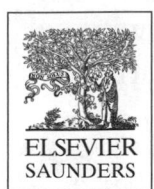

ELSEVIER
SAUNDERS

SAUNDERS
An Imprint of Elsevier

11830 Westline Industrial Drive
St. Louis, Missouri 63146

Instructor's Curriculum Resource to accompany
MEDICAL TERMINOLOGY: A SHORT COURSE, Fourth Edition   1-4160-2412-3
Copyright © 2005, 2003, 1999, 1991 by Elsevier Inc.

Previous editions copyrighted 2003, 1999, 1991

International Standard Book Number 1-4160-2412-3

Printed in the United States of America

Last digit is the print number: 9 8 7 6 5 4 3 2 1

Table of Contents

I. Introduction and Objectives

I'm pleased that you have chosen *Medical Terminology: A Short Course, Fourth Edition,* as the text for your medical terminology classes. I hope that you will enjoy using it with your students and that you will personally communicate any suggestions and comments to me as you teach your classes. My personal e-mail address is MedDavi@aol.com.

The Preface of the text explains the general format and purpose of the book. I will restate these objectives here, with our goals as teachers in mind.

1. To present a **concise, introductory** course in medical terminology that gives basic principles for understanding the language and an overview of terms from many areas of medicine.

2. To present the material in **easy-to-read** language, not assuming previous student knowledge of science or biology.

3. To provide extensive **written exercises** with **answers,** so students can check their answers and correct their mistakes. *Review Sheets and Pronunciation of Terms sections are given in each chapter* and can also be used as classroom exercises.

4. To include terms that are **practical** and commonly found in the day-to-day work of allied health personnel. Medical vignettes and practical applications are presented in each chapter, as well as in the Instructor's Manual.

5. To use dynamic **illustrations** to make the terminology come "alive" and to help the student visualize terms related to structure, function, and pathology.

6. To provide **reference** material for during and after the course is completed. Diagrams of body systems with combining forms, medical terms, pathology, laboratory tests, diagnostic and treatment procedures, and matching exercises *(Appendix I),* a list of Diagnostic Tests and Procedures *(Appendix II),* and Abbreviations, Symbols, and Acronyms *(Appendix III),* as well as three *Glossaries:* Medical Terms, Word Parts, and English to Spanish terms, help the student decipher medical language in the workplace.

II. Course Outlines

The text is intended for short (12- to 24-hour) medical terminology courses, as taught in hospitals, health maintenance organizations, adult education courses, and insurance companies. I have used the textual material in courses of varying lengths and have found that it can be easily adapted to different time frames. Below are some suggestions for use of the book in planning a medical terminology course. Actual time spent on each chapter will vary with the level and background of students in the class. I never rush through material just to cover it. Time should also be allotted for quizzes after each chapter is studied.

12- to 16-hour Course

Chapter 1	Basic Word Structure	3-4 hours
Chapter 2	Organization of the Body	3-4 hours
Chapter 3	Suffixes	3-4 hours
Chapter 4	Prefixes	3-4 hours

20- to 24-hour Course

Chapter 1	Basic Word Structure	3-4 hours
Chapter 2	Organization of the Body	3-4 hours
Chapter 3	Suffixes	3-4 hours
Chapter 4	Prefixes	3-4 hours
Chapter 5	Medical Specialists and Case Reports	2 hours
Appendix I	Body Systems	6 hours

III. Study Suggestions

I tell my students that if they attend class and complete and correct the exercises in the text at home, they will be successful in learning medical terminology. They must also **write** words **over** and **over** and test themselves by completing the reviews and pronunciation lists in each chapter. There is no substitute for that kind of study. Many of my students make flash cards to quiz themselves and thus review the material. One side of the card has the medical term and the other its meaning. Other students ask family members to test them on terms from the Pronunciation of Terms list or the Review Sheet in each chapter.

In class, I ask students to pronounce the terms on the Pronunciation of Terms list and then explain their meanings. This gives practice in both pronouncing and understanding the terms.

The expanded CD-ROM gives the student additional practice and instruction in medical terminology. A wide variety of types of questions, including matching, short answer, multiple choice, spelling bees, and diagrams to label, reinforce the information in the text. I suggest that you tell students to use the CD-ROM after completing the work in the book. Also, they can use the medical terminology glossary in the CD-ROM to hear the pronunciation of terms.

I give frequent quizzes, one after each chapter. Students find that tests help them focus on study of the material. Part IV of the Instructor's Manual includes several types of quizzes for each chapter:

- Multiple Choice Quizzes
- Spelling and Comprehension Quizzes. I routinely give these in my classes. They quickly and easily test a student's ability to spell terms on the Pronunciation of Terms list in each chapter, and also test the student's comprehension of the terms. Here's how they work: after each student has a copy of the quiz in front of himself or herself, you (the instructor) read aloud the list of "spelling words" provided in the appropriate answer key. Listening to your pronunciations, the students try to spell the words in the spaces provided on the quiz. Then, in the second part of the quiz, they match the words they just spelled with a list of meanings. The quiz ends with a relevant matching exercise.
- Review Quizzes. These quizzes are based on the review page in each chapter. The students should complete the reviews and then test their knowledge by covering one list, writing answers again, and reversing the process. The Review Quiz tests their knowledge of this important aspect of terminology.
- Crossword Puzzle Quizzes. These were designed by Kathy Trawick of Little Rock, Arkansas. Please let us know how your students like them and encourage your students to compose their own puzzles to share with us in the next edition.

The **Proficiency Exam** included on p. 83 of this manual may be used to test students who study the material (Chapters 1-5) on their own. It includes multiple choice, true/false, and short-answer questions.

If a student attends class and achieves a grade of C– or better on quizzes and the final exam, he or she successfully completes the course. Correcting a quiz or doing it again helps a student's grade.

My more complete textbook, *The Language of Medicine,* seventh edition, is a good reference for your teaching. It contains additional practical application examples throughout. In addition, the instructor's manual contains useful information to aid in teaching your course: teacher-tested suggestions and activities for individuals and groups, quizzes, explanations of diseases, and terminology. Try it!

Don't forget that I appreciate an ongoing dialog with instructors. My e-mail address is MedDavi@aol.com.

IV. Teaching Strategies, Class Activities, and Quizzes

Chapter 1

Basic Word Structure

This chapter introduces analysis of medical terms and builds a vocabulary of combining forms, suffixes, and prefixes. The student's goal is to understand how medical terms are broken down into component parts, not just to memorize terms and meanings. I introduce the subject matter by emphasizing three important objectives of the learning process:

A. Divide words into component parts and learn the meanings of the parts so that when totally new terms are encountered they can be understood.

B. Relate the terms to understanding where the organs are located and how they function in health and disease. My teaching focuses on explaining the terminology in relation to how the body works.

C. Concentrate on spelling and pronouncing words correctly.

I begin teaching Chapter 1 by giving examples of how medical terms are broken into component parts. Students suggest terms, and I show them how to divide the terms into roots, suffixes, prefixes, combining vowels, and combining forms.

Next, I turn to the list of combining forms, suffixes, and prefixes (Section II) and explain the terms on the list. I relate the terms to the anatomy and physiology of the body. For example, for the term ADENOMA, I talk about glands and the differences between endocrine and exocrine glands. I keep the explanations simple, realizing that my students may not have backgrounds in biology or science. I also frequently ask questions in class to find out what is understood.

You will notice repetition of terms in the text. This reinforces the learning process and builds student confidence as she or he recognizes familiar terminology.

A new addition to this chapter in this edition is a table on formations of plurals. Use it early on to help students learn these rules and apply them throughout the course.

Included on the following pages are exercises that can be photocopied to use in class as you teach the terms in the first chapter. The answers to the exercises are found on p. 17.

Matching Exercises

A.   Match the combining form in Column I with its meaning in Column II.

Column I		Column II
1. aden/o	_____	A. head
2. arthr/o	_____	B. urinary bladder
3. bi/o	_____	C. heart
4. carcin/o	_____	D. joint
5. cardi/o	_____	E. skin
6. cephal/o	_____	F. gland
7. cerebr/o	_____	G. cell
8. cyst/o	_____	H. brain (largest part)
9. cyt/o	_____	I. cancerous
10. dermat/o	_____	J. life

B.   Match the combining form in Column I with its meaning in Column II.

Column I		Column II
1. electr/o	_____	A. intestines (usually small intestine)
2. encephal/o	_____	B. blood
3. enter/o	_____	C. stomach
4. erythr/o	_____	D. brain
5. gastr/o	_____	E. liver
6. gnos/o	_____	F. abdomen
7. gynec/o	_____	G. red
8. hemat/o	_____	H. electricity
9. hepat/o	_____	I. knowledge
10. lapar/o	_____	J. woman, female

C.   Match the combining form in Column I with its meaning in Column II.

Column I		Column II
1. leuk/o	_____	A. disease
2. nephr/o, ren/o	_____	B. bone
3. neur/o	_____	C. white
4. onc/o	_____	D. flesh
5. ophthalm/o	_____	E. tumor
6. oste/o	_____	F. nose
7. path/o	_____	G. nerve
8. psych/o	_____	H. clot
9. rhin/o	_____	I. kidney
10. sarc/o	_____	J. eye
11. thromb/o	_____	K. mind

D.   Match the suffix in Column I with its meaning in Column II.

Column I		Column II
1. -al, -ic	_____	A. inflammation
2. -algia	_____	B. cell
3. -cyte	_____	C. process of study
4. -ectomy	_____	D. removal, excision
5. -emia	_____	E. record
6. -gram	_____	F. specialist in the study of
7. -ism	_____	G. pertaining to
8. -itis	_____	H. condition; process
9. -logist	_____	I. pain
10. -logy	_____	J. blood condition
11. -oma	_____	K. state of
12. -osis	_____	L. tumor, mass
13. -scope	_____	M. instrument to visually examine
14. -scopy	_____	N. abnormal condition
15. -sis	_____	O. process of cutting; incision
16. -tomy	_____	P. process of visual examination

E.   Match the prefix in Column I with its meaning in Column II.

Column I		Column II
1. a-, an-	_____	A. behind
2. dia-	_____	B. across, through
3. endo-	_____	C. outside
4. exo-	_____	D. below, less than normal
5. hyper-	_____	E. within
6. hypo-	_____	F. no, not
7. pro-	_____	G. before
8. re-	_____	H. complete, thorough
9. retro-	_____	I. too much, excessive
10. trans-	_____	J. back

Synonymous Word Parts

Since students notice that there may be two combining forms for the same organ or part of the body (both REN/O and NEPHR/O mean "kidney"), they often ask which combining form is used with a particular suffix. I have given a general explanation in the text (under REN/O). The *Glossary of Word Parts* (English to Medical Terms) gives the student further guidance in this regard. Included below is a list of organs and body parts that have two combining forms and examples of terms that illustrate the use of each.

Organ or Body Part	Combining Form	Combining Form
abdomen	abdomin/o (abdominal)	lapar/o (laparoscopy)
backbone	vertebr/o (vertebral)	spondyl/o (spondylitis)
bladder (urinary)	vesic/o (vesical)	cyst/o (cystitis)
blood vessel	vas/o (vasoconstriction)	angi/o (angiogram)
breast	mamm/o (mammogram)	mast/o (mastectomy)
eardrum	tympan/o (tympanic)	myring/o (myringotomy)
eye	ocul/o (ocular)	ophthalm/o (ophthalmoscope)
heart	coron/o (coronary)	cardi/o (cardiology)
kidney	ren/o (renal)	nephr/o (nephritis)
lung	pulmon/o (pulmonary)	pneumon/o (pneumonectomy)
mouth	or/o (oral)	stomat/o (stomatitis)
muscle	muscul/o (muscular)	my/o (myoma)
nose	nas/o (nasal)	rhin/o (rhinitis)
ovary	ovari/o (ovarian)	oophor/o (oophorectomy)
skin	cutane/o (cutaneous)	dermat/o (dermatitis)
uterus	uter/o (uterine)	hyster/o (hysterectomy)
vagina	vagin/o (vaginal)	colp/o (colposcopy)
vein	ven/o (venous)	phleb/o (phlebitis)

Chapter 1 Multiple Choice Quiz

1. A combining form is:
   - A. the word ending
   - B. the root plus combining vowel
   - C. the prefix
   - D. the prefix plus combining vowel
   - E. the root and suffix

2. The combining form meaning "joint" is:
   - A. aden/o
   - B. -itis
   - C. -algia
   - D. arthr/o
   - E. oste/o

3. A suffix meaning "inflammation" is:
   - A. -itis
   - B. -osis
   - C. -ac
   - D. -al
   - E. -tomy

4. A prefix meaning "under," "deficient," or "less than normal" is:
   - A. re-
   - B. hyper-
   - C. trans-
   - D. -emia
   - E. hypo-

5. A suffix meaning "study of" is:
   - A. -pathy
   - B. -logy
   - C. -gram
   - D. -scopy
   - E. -osis

6. Tumor of a gland:
   - A. arthrosis
   - B. arthroscope
   - C. adenoma
   - D. nephroma
   - E. hepatitis

7. Visual examination of the urinary bladder:
   - A. cystoscopy
   - B. cytology
   - C. cystogram
   - D. nephroscopy
   - E. cystoscope

8. Prediction about the outcome of treatment:
   - A. prognosis
   - B. psychosis
   - C. diagnosis
   - D. biopsy
   - E. pathology

9. Nerve pain:
   - A. neural
   - B. arthralgia
   - C. cephalgia
   - D. nueralgia
   - E. neuralgia

10. Ren/o and nephr/o both mean:
    - A. heart
    - B. liver
    - C. blood
    - D. kidney
    - E. intestine

11. Which term relates to the brain?
    - A. anemia
    - B. cerebral
    - C. rhinitis
    - D. thrombosis
    - E. gastrotomy

12. A cancerous tumor is a(an):
    - A. hematoma
    - B. adenoma
    - C. oncology
    - D. gastralgia
    - E. carcinoma

13. A red blood cell:
    - A. platelet
    - B. thrombocyte
    - C. erythrocyte
    - D. leukocyte
    - E. resection

14. A cerebrovascular accident (CVA) can be caused by:
    - A. gastritis
    - B. osteitis
    - C. adenosis
    - D. dermatitis
    - E. thrombosis

15. An instrument to visually examine the urinary bladder is called a(an):
    A. cystoscopy
    B. cystoscope
    C. gastroscope
    D. arthroscopy
    E. excision

16. Excessive (more than normal) amount of sugar in the blood is called:
    A. hypothyroidism
    B. hyperthyroidism
    C. hyperglycemia
    D. hypoglycemia
    E. hypodermic

17. A gastrectomy is a(an):
    A. gastric resection
    B. gastroscopy
    C. visual examination of the abdomen
    D. incision of the stomach
    E. incision of a gland

18. Glands that secrete hormones are:
    A. enteral
    B. endocrine
    C. exocrine
    D. adenomas
    E. neural glands

19. Cancerous condition of white blood cells with high numbers of immature cells:
    A. leukemia
    B. anemia
    C. adenosis
    D. hepatoma
    E. osteoma

20. Incision of the abdomen:
    A. laparoscopy
    B. rhinotomy
    C. laparotomy
    D. gastrotomy
    E. gastroscopy

21. A malignant (cancerous) tumor of flesh tissue:
    A. carcinoma
    B. sarcoma
    C. neuroma
    D. hepatoma
    E. nephroma

22. A doctor who performs autopsies and examines biopsy samples:
    A. oncologist
    B. gynecologist
    C. hematologist
    D. endocrinologist
    E. pathologist

23. A record of the electricity in the brain:
    A. arthrogram
    B. electrocardiogram
    C. resection
    D. electroencephalogram
    E. nephrectomy

24. Inflammation of the small intestine:
    A. osteitis
    B. hepatitis
    C. rhinitis
    D. adenitis
    E. enteritis

25. Blood protein found in red blood cells:
    A. sarcoma
    B. hemoglobin
    C. hematoma
    D. erythrocyte
    E. hepatoma

12

Chapter 1   Spelling and Comprehension Quiz

I. Spelling

1. _____   11. _____

2. _____   12. _____

3. _____   13. _____

4. _____   14. _____

5. _____   15. _____

6. _____   16. _____

7. _____   17. _____

8. _____   18. _____

9. _____   19. _____

10. _____   20. _____

II. Comprehension: Match the terms listed above with their meanings below.

_____ white blood cell

_____ collection (mass) of blood

_____ inflammation of bone

_____ visual examination of the urinary bladder

_____ inflammation of the small intestine

_____ specialist in women's diseases

_____ high blood sugar

_____ incision of a nerve

_____ benign tumor of a gland

_____ condition of low level of hormone secreted by a gland in the neck

_____ red blood cell

_____ pertaining to through the urethra

_____ resection of a kidney

_____ removal of living tissue and examination under a microscope

_____ abnormal condition of the mind

_____ pain of a joint

_____ pertaining to under the liver

_____ cancerous tumor of connective (flesh) tissue

_____ deficiency of red blood cells or amount of hemoglobin in the red blood cells

_____ platelet; clotting cell

14

III. Matching: Match the combining form in Column I with its meaning in Column II.

Column I		Column II
1. ophthalm/o	_____	A. abdomen
2. gastr/o	_____	B. brain
3. onc/o	_____	C. joint
4. cephal/o	_____	D. nose
5. rhin/o	_____	E. eye
6. aden/o	_____	F. disease
7. lapar/o	_____	G. stomach
8. arthr/o	_____	H. head
9. path/o	_____	I. gland
10. encephal/o	_____	J. tumor

Chapter 1   Review Quiz

I. Give meanings for the following combining forms:

1. cyt/o _____

2. rhin/o _____

3. hemat/o _____

4. glyc/o _____

5. aden/o _____

6. oste/o _____

7. arthr/o _____

8. thromb/o _____

9. lapar/o _____

10. cephal/o _____

11. nephr/o _____

II. Give combining forms for the following English words:

1. urinary bladder _____

2. nerve _____

3. liver _____

4. eye _____

5. woman, female _____

6. white _____

7. red _____

8. disease _____

9. stomach _____

10. small intestine _____

11. heart _____

12. mind _____

III. Give meanings for the following suffixes:

1. -ectomy _____

2. -oma _____

3. -logy _____

4. -emia _____

5. -tomy _____

6. -globin _____

7. -algia _____

8. -itis _____

9. -osis _____

10. -scopy _____

11. -scope _____

IV. Give meanings for the following prefixes:

1. hyper- _____

2. sub- _____

3. trans- _____

4. endo- _____

5. pro- _____

6. hypo- _____

7. retro- _____

8. exo- _____

9. dia- _____

10. dys- _____

11. a-, an- _____

12. aut- _____

Chapter 1 Crossword Puzzle Quiz

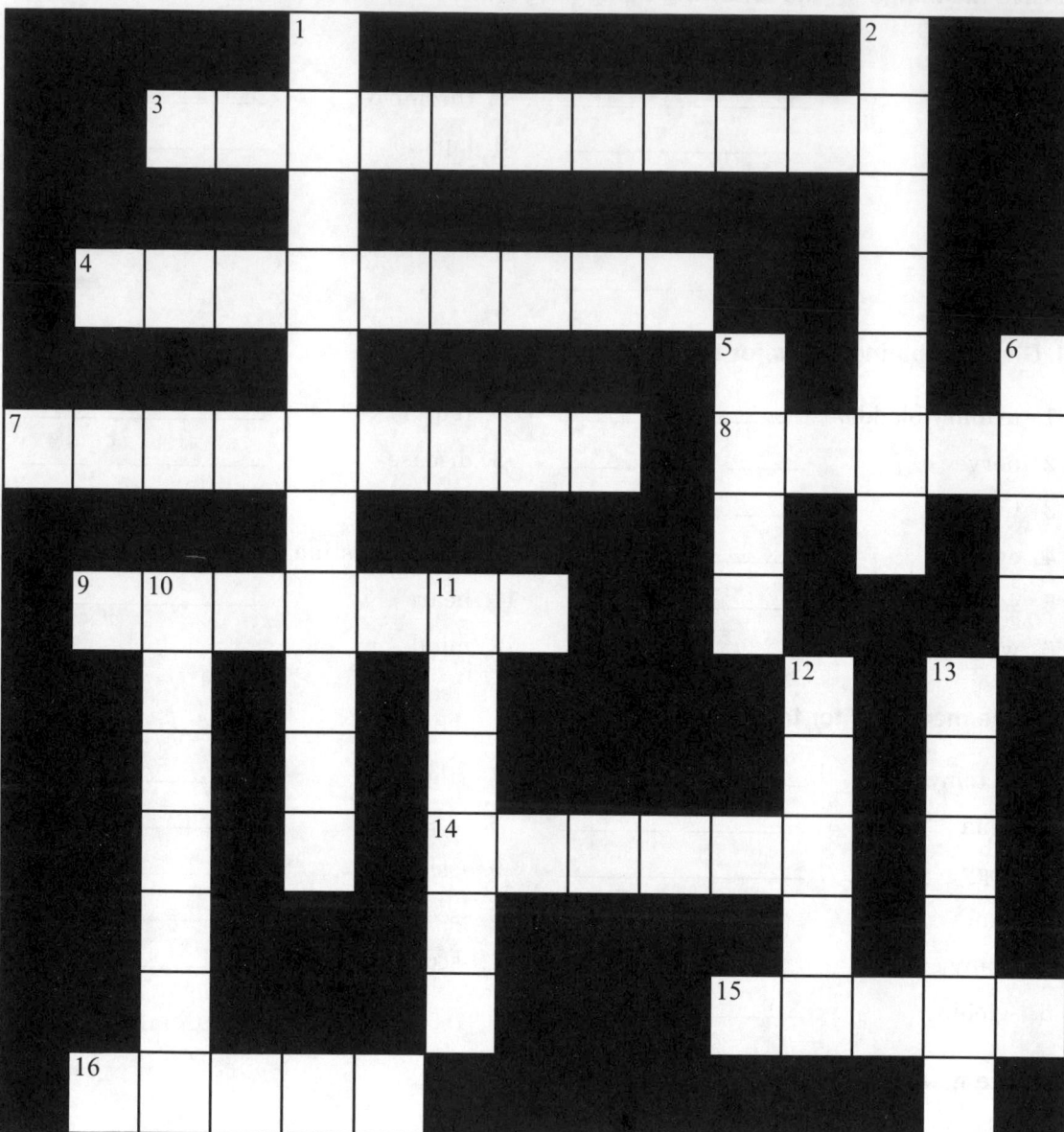

Across

3. a clotting cell
4. abnormal condition of the kidney
7. incision or cut into a nerve
8. combining form meaning *bone*
9. combining form meaning *cancer*
14. combining form meaning *liver*
15. prefix meaning *back* or *behind*
16. combining form meaning *disease*

Down

1. process of visual examination of a joint
2. combining form meaning *skin*
5. suffix meaning *study of*
6. suffix meaning *cut into* or *incision*
10. tumor (benign) of a gland
11. combining form meaning *kidney*
12. suffix meaning *instrument to view*
13. combining form meaning *small intestine*

Chapter 1   Answers

Matching Exercises

A. 1. F   6. A
    2. D   7. H
    3. J   8. B
    4. I   9. G
    5. C   10. E

B. 1. H   6. I
    2. D   7. J
    3. A   8. B
    4. G   9. E
    5. C   10. F

C. 1. C   7. A
    2. I   8. K
    3. G   9. F
    4. E   10. D
    5. J   11. H
    6. B

D. 1. G   9. F
    2. I   10. C
    3. C   11. L
    4. D   12. N
    5. J   13. M
    6. E   14. P
    7. H   15. K
    8. A   16. O

E. 1. F   6. D
    2. H   7. G
    3. E   8. J
    4. C   9. A
    5. I   10. B

Multiple Choice

  1. B   14. E
  2. D   15. B
  3. A   16. C
  4. E   17. A
  5. B   18. B
  6. C   19. A
  7. A   20. C
  8. A   21. B
  9. E   22. E
 10. D   23. D
 11. B   24. E
 12. E   25. B
 13. C

Spelling and Comprehension Quiz

I. Spelling

1. adenoma
2. anemia
3. arthralgia
4. biopsy
5. cystoscopy
6. enteritis
7. erythrocyte
8. gynecologist
9. hematoma
10. hyperglycemia
11. hypothyroidism
12. leukocyte
13. nephrectomy
14. neurotomy
15. osteitis
16. psychosis
17. sarcoma
18. subhepatic
19. thrombocyte
20. transurethral

II. Comprehension

12   white blood cell
 9   collection (mass) of blood
15   inflammation of bone
 5   visual examination of the urinary bladder
 6   inflammation of the small intestine
 8   specialist in women's diseases
10   high blood sugar
14   incision of a nerve
 1   benign tumor of a gland
11   condition of low level of hormone secreted by a gland in the neck
 7   red blood cell
20   pertaining to through the urethra
13   resection of a kidney
 4   removal of living tissue and examination under a microscope
16   abnormal condition of the mind
 3   pain of a joint
18   pertaining to under the liver
17   cancerous tumor of connective (flesh) tissue
 2   deficiency of red blood cells or amount of hemoglobin in red blood cells
19   platelet; clotting cell

III. Matching

1. E
2. G
3. J
4. H
5. D
6. I
7. A
8. C
9. F
10. B

Review Quiz

I. 1. cell
2. nose
3. blood
4. sugar
5. gland
6. bone
7. joint
8. clot
9. abdomen
10. head
11. kidney

II. 1. cyst/o
2. neur/o
3. hepat/o
4. ophthalm/o
5. gynec/o
6. leuk/o
7. erythr/o
8. path/o
9. gastr/o
10. enter/o
11. cardi/o
12. psych/o

III. 1. removal, excision, resection
2. tumor; mass
3. study of
4. blood condition
5. process of cutting, incision
6. protein
7. pain
8. inflammation
9. abnormal condition
10. process of visual examination
11. instrument to visually examine

IV.
1. too much, above
2. under, below
3. across, through
4. in, within
5. before; forward
6. below, too little, deficient
7. behind
8. out, outside
9. complete; through
10. bad, painful, difficult, abnormal
11. no, not
12. self

Crossword Puzzle Quiz

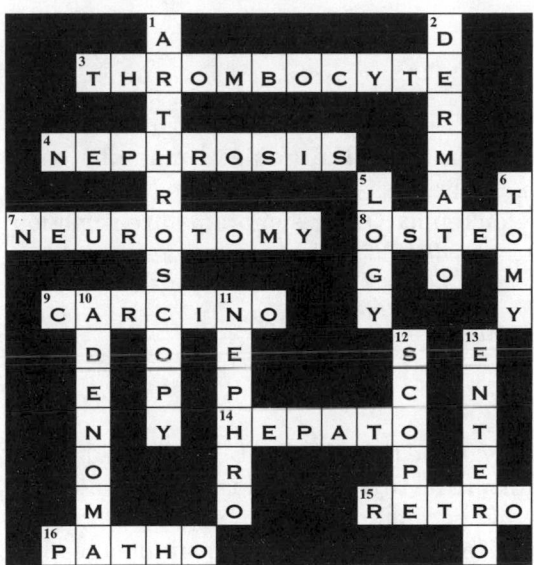

Dictation Sentences

Medical terms that are in **bold** are found in the chapter. Italicized terms may be new to students. Their definitions follow the paragraph.

1. Osteoarthritis

Osteoarthritis involves degeneration of the tissue within a joint. Loss of *cartilage* occurs, and bones thicken around the joint. **Arthralgia** is present. Involvement of the *pelvis,* knee, or *spine* causes more disability than osteoarthritis of other areas. X-rays and **arthroscopy** are helpful in **diagnosis** of the condition.

> *Cartilage: flexible connective tissue at the joint*
> *Pelvis: bones of the hip area*
> *Spine: backbone*

2. Leukemia

Leukemia is a disease of the blood marked by extremely high numbers of abnormal **leukocytes.** The condition begins in the *bone marrow,* and **diagnosis** is made by bone marrow **biopsy.** Symptoms include weakness and shortness of breath caused by too few **erythrocytes.** This **anemia** is secondary to the leukemia. Other symptoms are infection and fever caused by a deficiency of normal white blood cells and bleeding caused by low **platelet** levels.

> *Bone marrow: inner section of bone, containing developing blood cells*

3. Hyperthyroidism

Hyperthyroidism is a condition of increased activity of the thyroid gland. The thyroid gland is an **endocrine** gland in the neck. In hyperthyroidism, the thyroid gland is usually enlarged and secretes a greater-than-normal amount of thyroid hormone. Nervousness, *exophthalmos,* weight loss, *palpitations,* and *fatigue* often develop. Untreated hyperthyroidism may lead to **cardiac** failure and death.

> *Exophthalmos: swelling of tissue behind the eyeball*
> *Fatigue: tiredness*
> *Palpitations: pounding or racing of the heart*

Chapter 2

Organization of the Body

This chapter teaches terms that describe the organization of the body, the body cavities and organs therein, the divisions of the back, and the planes of the body. There is no attempt to teach terminology related to each individual system of the body in this chapter. Students, however, should consult the diagrams in *Appendix I* to locate organs in the different body systems. If time permits, after teaching Chapters 3, 4, and 5, you may wish to cover the systems of the body, including names of organs, descriptions, and combining forms, pathology laboratory tests, and procedures. See the material included for *Appendix I* later in this manual.

As you teach, a model of a human torso and a skeleton are useful to show students where organs are located. Included below is a list of organs and the body system to which each belongs. This list can be used by students to locate an organ in the systems diagrams of *Appendix I*.

Organs and Systems

Organ	System
adrenal glands	endocrine
anus	digestive
aorta	circulatory
appendix	digestive
arteries	circulatory
blood vessels	circulatory
bone marrow	musculoskeletal
brain	nervous
bronchial tubes	respiratory
capillaries	circulatory
carpals	musculoskeletal
cartilage	musculoskeletal
cerebellum	nervous
cerebrum	nervous
cervix	female reproductive
clavicle	musculoskeletal
coccyx	musculoskeletal
colon	digestive
cornea	sense organ (eye)
dermis	skin
diaphragm	musculoskeletal and respiratory
duodenum	digestive
ear	sense organ
epidermis	skin
esophagus	digestive
eye	sense organ
femur	musculoskeletal
fibula	musculoskeletal
gallbladder	digestive
heart	circulatory
humerus	musculoskeletal
ileum	digestive
ilium	musculoskeletal
jejunum	digestive
kidneys	urinary
larynx	respiratory
ligament	musculoskeletal
liver	digestive
lungs	respiratory
lymph nodes	circulatory (immune system)
medulla oblongata	nervous
meninges	nervous
metacarpals	musculoskeletal

Organ	System
metatarsals	musculoskeletal
nose	respiratory
optic nerve	sense organ and nervous
ovaries	female reproductive and endocrine
pancreas	digestive and endocrine
parathyroid glands	endocrine
patella	musculoskeletal
pelvis	musculoskeletal
phalanges	musculoskeletal
pharynx	digestive and respiratory
pituitary gland	endocrine
pleura	respiratory
prostate gland	male reproductive
rectum	digestive
renal pelvis	urinary
retina	sense organ (eye)
ribs	musculoskeletal
sacrum	musculoskeletal
scapula	musculoskeletal
sclera	sense organ (eye)
scrotum	male reproductive
sigmoid colon	digestive
spinal column	musculoskeletal
spinal cord	nervous
sternum	musculoskeletal
sweat gland	skin
tarsals	musculoskeletal
tendon	musculoskeletal
testes	male reproductive
thyroid gland	endocrine
tibia	musculoskeletal
trachea	respiratory
tympanic membrane	sense organ (ear)
ureter	urinary
urethra	urinary
urinary bladder	urinary
uterus	female reproductive
vagina	female reproductive
veins	circulatory
vena cava	circulatory

Matching Exercises for Organs and Systems

I. Write a system next to the organ or body structure that is included in that system. Sometimes more than one system may be written. Write the common name of the organ in the parentheses wherever indicated.

Systems

cardiovascular   musculoskeletal

digestive   nervous

endocrine   respiratory

female reproductive   skin and sense organs

lymphatic   urinary

male reproductive

Organ or Structure

1. brain _____
2. femur (   ) _____
3. anus _____
4. cartilage _____
5. aorta _____
6. bronchial tubes _____
7. coccyx (   ) _____
8. carpals (   ) _____
9. cervix _____
10. adrenals _____

II. Write a system next to the organ or body structure that is included in that system. Sometimes more than one system may be written. Write the common name of the organ in the parentheses wherever indicated.

Systems

cardiovascular   musculoskeletal

digestive   nervous

endocrine   respiratory

female reproductive   skin and sense organs

lymphatic   urinary

male reproductive

Organ or Structure

1. ileum _____
2. gallbladder _____
3. kidney _____
4. larynx (   ) _____
5. ilium _____
6. meninges _____
7. epidermis _____
8. diaphragm _____
9. cornea _____
10. ligament _____

III. Write a system next to the organ or body structure that is included in that system. Sometimes more than one system may be written. Write the common name of the organ in the parentheses wherever indicated.

Systems

cardiovascular	musculoskeletal
digestive	nervous
endocrine	respiratory
female reproductive	skin and sense organs
lymphatic	urinary
male reproductive	

Organ or Structure

1. metatarsals ( )_____
2. patella ( )_____
3. pharynx ( )_____
4. pancreas_____
5. renal pelvis_____
6. retina_____
7. pelvis_____
8. scapula ( )_____
9. spinal cord_____
10. spinal column_____

IV. Write a system next to the organ or body structure that is Included in that system. Sometimes more than one system may be written. Write the common name of the organ in the parentheses wherever indicated.

Systems

cardiovascular	musculoskeletal
digestive	nervous
endocrine	respiratory
female reproductive	skin and sense organs
lymphatic	urinary
male reproductive	

Organ or Structure

1. sigmoid colon_____
2. testes_____
3. sweat gland_____
4. tibia ( )_____
5. thyroid gland_____

6. trachea ( )_____

7. tympanic membrane_____

8. uterus_____

9. vein_____

10. ureter_____

11. vena cava_____

12. sternum ( )_____

13. prostate gland_____

14. pleura_____

15. phalanges ( )_____

Chapter 2 Multiple Choice Quiz

1. The system that controls breathing is the:
   A. circulatory system
   B. digestive system
   C. nervous system
   D. endocrine system
   E. respiratory system

2. The individual unit that each part of the body is composed of is called a(an):
   A. organ
   B. cell
   C. tissue
   D. system
   E. gland

3. The system that supports the body and allows it to move is the:
   A. skin and sense organs
   B. nervous system
   C. urinary system
   D. musculoskeletal system
   E. female reproductive system

4. The voice box is the:
   A. larynx
   B. pharynx
   C. trachea
   D. esophagus
   E. bronchial tube

5. The tube leading from the bladder to the outside of the body is the:
   A. urethra
   B. uterus
   C. large intestine
   D. vagina
   E. ureter

6. The endocrine gland located at the base of the brain is the:
   A. adrenal gland
   B. prostate gland
   C. pituitary gland
   D. thyroid gland
   E. pancreas

7. The nervous tissue that is surrounded by backbones is the:
   A. vertebrae
   B. spinal column
   C. spinal cord
   D. pelvis
   E. brain

8. The chest cavity is the:
   A. cranial cavity
   B. abdominal cavity
   C. spinal cavity
   D. pelvic cavity
   E. thoracic cavity

9. The membrane surrounding the organs in the abdomen is the:
   A. peritoneum
   B. esophagus
   C. pleura
   D. diaphragm
   E. mediastinum

10. The bones in the region of the hip:
    A. trachea
    B. carpals
    C. cervix
    D. pelvis
    E. phalanges

11. The space in the chest that contains the heart and other organs is the:
    A. mediastinum
    B. pleural cavity
    C. cranial cavity
    D. abdomen
    E. spinal cavity

12. A backbone is a(an):
    A. disk
    B. vertebra
    C. cartilage
    D. vertebrae
    E. spinal nerve

13. The backbones in the region of the neck are:
   A. lumbar bones
   B. cervical bones
   C. coccygeal bones
   D. thoracic bones
   E. sacral bones

14. Flexible connective tissue found between bones at joints is:
   A. nervous tissue
   B. muscle tissue
   C. skin
   D. cartilage
   E. epithelial tissue

15. The tailbone is the:
   A. sacrum
   B. coccyx
   C. pharynx
   D. larynx
   E. cartilage

16. Anterior means:
   A. side
   B. back
   C. front
   D. lateral
   E. posterior

17. The plane that divides the body into a right and left side is:
   A. sagittal
   B. frontal
   C. transverse
   D. cervical
   E. sacral

18. A series of x-ray images that show the body in cross-section is:
   A. MRI (magnetic resonance imaging)
   B. chest x-rays
   C. gastroscopy
   D. laparoscopy
   E. CT scan (computerized tomography)

19. Pertaining to skin cells:
   A. lumbar
   B. vertebral
   C. cervical
   D. esophageal
   E. epithelial

20. Incision of the skull:
   A. laparotomy
   B. craniotomy
   C. laryngectomy
   D. rhinotomy
   E. tracheotomy

21. Pertaining to the throat:
   A. thoracic
   B. esophageal
   C. pharyngeal
   D. tracheal
   E. laryngeal

22. Inflammation of the membrane surrounding the lungs:
   A. pleuritis
   B. bronchitis
   C. lateral
   D. pleural
   E. rhinitis

23. The transverse plane:
   A. shows a side view of the body
   B. divides the body into front and back portions
   C. divides the body into upper and lower portions
   D. divides the body into right and left parts
   E. cannot be viewed with a CT scan

24. Visual examination of the abdomen by making a small incision near the navel is called:
   A. laparoscope
   B. laparotomy
   C. mediastinoscopy
   D. laparoscopy
   E. epithelial biopsy

Chapter 2   Spelling and Comprehension Quiz

I. Spelling

1. _____   11. _____

2. _____   12. _____

3. _____   13. _____

4. _____   14. _____

5. _____   15. _____

6. _____   16. _____

7. _____   17. _____

8. _____   18. _____

9. _____   19. _____

10. _____   20. _____

II. Comprehension: Match the terms listed above with their meanings below.

_____ pertaining to the tube leading from the throat to the stomach

_____ visual examination of the tube leading from the windpipe to the lungs

_____ incision of the chest

_____ flexible, connective tissue near joints

_____ pertaining to the area between the lungs in the chest

_____ throat

_____ muscle separating the abdominal and chest cavities

_____ incision of the skull

_____ pertaining to the side

_____ inflammation of the liver

_____ pertaining to the lower back region (loin)

_____ pertaining to the front

_____ an endocrine organ at the base of the brain

_____ pertaining to the membrane surrounding the abdomen

_____ incision of the abdomen

_____ inflammation of the membrane surrounding the lungs

_____ a backbone

_____ pertaining to the neck

_____ female organ that holds and provides nourishment for developing fetus

_____ pertaining to cells that cover the skin and line internal organs

III. Match the combining form in Column I with its meaning in Column II.

Column I		Column II
1. ureter	_____	A. tailbone
2. spinal column	_____	B. bones of the hip
3. larynx	_____	C. all the bones of the back
4. spinal cord	_____	D. pad of tissue separating backbones
5. urethra	_____	E. voice box
6. trachea	_____	F. nervous tissue connected to the brain
7. coccyx	_____	G. five fused backbones below the waist
8. pelvis	_____	H. tube from the kidney to the bladder
9. disk (disc)	_____	I. windpipe
10. sacrum	_____	J. tube from bladder to outside of body

Chapter 2   Review Quiz

I. Give meanings for the following combining forms:

1. cervic/o _____
2. coccyg/o _____
3. crani/o _____
4. anter/o _____
5. bronch/o _____
6. thorac/o _____
7. hepat/o _____
8. pleur/o _____
9. pharyng/o _____
10. trache/o _____

11. later/o _____
12. lapar/o _____
13. laryng/o _____
14. peritone/o _____
15. mediastin/o _____
16. pelv/o _____
17. abdomin/o _____
18. sacr/o _____
19. poster/o _____
20. epitheli/o _____

II. Give suffixes for the following English words:

1. tumor or mass _____
2. removal _____
3. inflammation _____
4. incision _____
5. cell _____
6. process of visually examining _____
7. process of study _____

Chapter 2   Crossword Puzzle Quiz

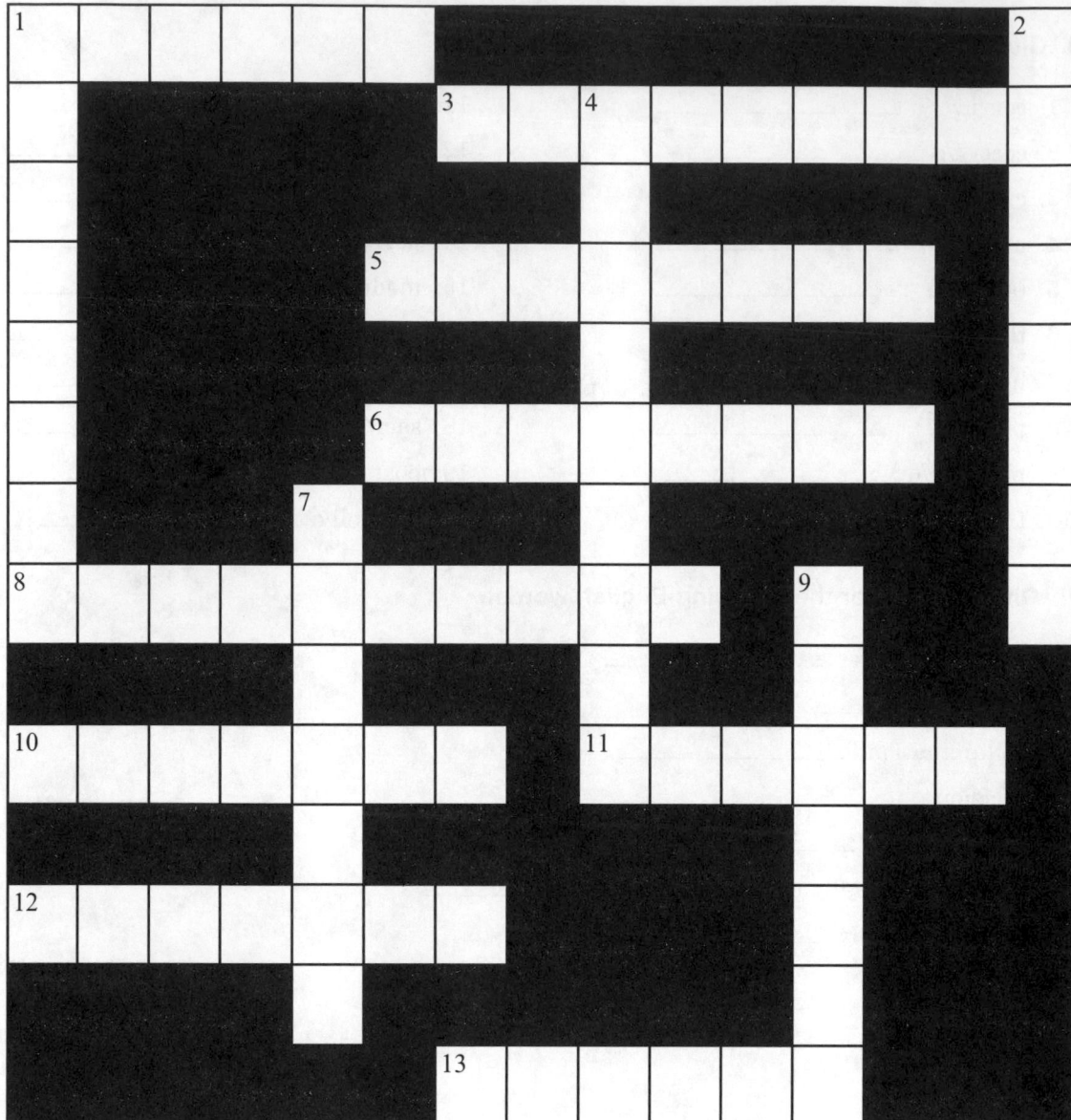

Across

1. combining form meaning *skull*
3. inflammation of the liver
5. *front* part of the body
6. combining form meaning *throat*
8. a lymph cell
10. pertaining to the side
11. pertaining to five fused bones in the lower back
12. combining form meaning *bronchial tube*
13. combining form meaning *abdomen*

Down

1. pertaining to the neck
2. combining form meaning *tube leading from the throat to the stomach*
4. inflammation of the membrane surrounding the lungs
7. combining form meaning *chest*
9. combining form meaning *voice box*

Chapter 2   Answers

Matching Exercises for Organs and Systems

I. 1. nervous
2. (thigh bone) musculoskeletal
3. digestive
4. musculoskeletal
5. cardiovascular

6. respiratory
7. (tailbone) musculoskeletal
8. (wrist bones) musculoskeletal
9. female reproductive
10. endocrine

II. 1. digestive
2. digestive
3. urinary
4. (voice box) respiratory
5. musculoskeletal

6. nervous
7. skin and sense organs
8. respiratory
9. skin and sense organs
10. musculoskeletal

III. 1. (foot bones) musculoskeletal
2. (knee bone) musculoskeletal
3. (throat) digestive
4. digestive and endocrine
5. urinary

6. skin and sense organs
7. musculoskeletal
8. (shoulder bone) musculoskeletal
9. nervous
10. musculoskeletal

IV. 1. digestive
2. male reproductive
3. skin and sense organs
4. (shin bone) musculoskeletal
5. endocrine
6. (windpipe) respiratory
7. skin and sense organs
8. female reproductive

9. cardiovascular
10. urinary
11. cardiovascular
12. (breast bone) musculoskeletal
13. male reproductive
14. respiratory
15. (finger and toe bones) musculoskeletal

Multiple Choice Quiz

1. E
2. B
3. D
4. A
5. A
6. C
7. C
8. E
9. A
10. D
11. A
12. B
13. B
14. D
15. B
16. C
17. A
18. E
19. E
20. B
21. C
22. A
23. C
24. D

Spelling and Comprehension Quiz

I. Spelling

1. anterior
2. bronchoscopy
3. cartilage
4. cervical
5. craniotomy
6. diaphragm
7. epithelial
8. esophageal
9. hepatitis
10. laparotomy
11. lateral
12. lumbar
13. mediastinal
14. peritoneal
15. pharynx
16. pituitary gland
17. pleuritis
18. thoracotomy
19. uterus
20. vertebra

II. Comprehension

8 pertaining to the tube leading from the throat to the stomach
2 visual examination of the tube leading from the windpipe to the lungs
18 incision of the chest
3 flexible connective tissue near joints
13 pertaining to the area between the lungs in the chest
15 throat
6 muscle separating the abdominal and chest cavities
5 incision of the skull
11 pertaining to the side
9 inflammation of the liver
12 pertaining to the lower back region (loin)
1 pertaining to the front
16 an endocrine organ at the base of the brain
14 pertaining to the membrane surrounding the abdomen
10 incision of the abdomen
17 inflammation of the membrane surrounding the lungs
20 a backbone
4 pertaining to the neck
19 female organ that holds and provides nourishment for the developing fetus
7 pertaining to cells that cover the skin and line internal organs

III. Matching

1. H
2. C
3. E
4. F
5. J
6. I
7. A
8. B
9. D
10. G

Review Quiz

I. 1. neck
   2. coccyx (tailbone)
   3. skull
   4. front
   5. bronchial tubes
   6. chest
   7. liver
   8. pleura
   9. throat (pharynx)
   10. trachea (windpipe)
   11. side
   12. abdomen
   13. larynx (voice box)
   14. peritoneum
   15. mediastinum

16. bones of the hip
17. abdomen
18. sacrum
19. back (of body); behind
20. skin

II. 1. -oma
2. -ectomy
3. -itis
4. -tomy
5. -cyte
6. -scopy
7. -logy

Crossword Puzzle Quiz

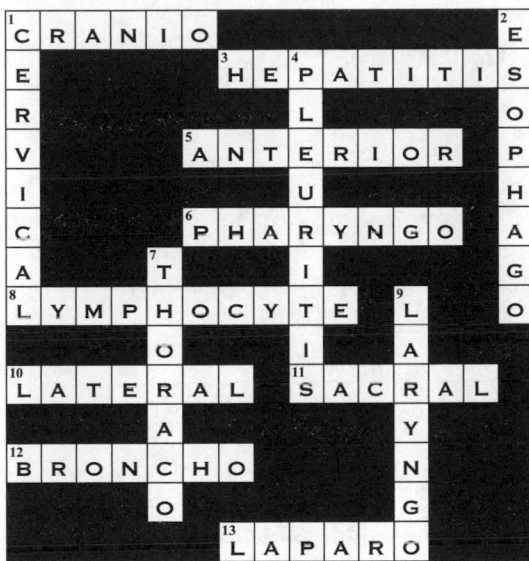

Dictation Sentences

Medical terms that are in **bold** are found in the chapter. Italicized terms may be new to students. Their definitions follow the paragraph.

1. Hepatitis

Hepatitis is inflammation of the liver. Most often, it occurs by viral infection. Hepatitis A, caused by the hepatitis A virus, is spread by direct contact through food or water contaminated by *feces*. Hepatitis B is caused by the hepatitis B virus. This virus is spread by blood transfusions that contain the virus or by use of contaminated needles and instruments. Hepatitis C is transmitted by blood transfusions or by *percutaneous* infection when *intravenous* drug users share needles.

> *Feces: solid wastes eliminated from the body via the rectum and anus*
> *Intravenous: pertaining to within a vein*
> *Percutaneous: pertaining to through (per-) the skin (cutane/o)*

2. Pleuritis

Pleuritis is also known as pleurisy. It is inflammation of the **pleura** surrounding the lungs. Symptoms are painful breathing, known as *dyspnea,* and pain in the chest, called *pleurodynia.* Part of the pleura near the **diaphragm** may be affected, and pain may extend to the **abdomen.** When fluid accumulates in the pleural cavity, it is a **pleural** *effusion.*

> *Dyspnea: painful (dys-) breathing (-pnea)*
> *Effusion: escape of fluid into a space such as the pleural cavity*
> *Pleurodynia: pain (-dynia) in the chest (pleur/o here indicates the chest wall)*

3. Mediastinum

The **mediastinum** is a part of the **thoracic** cavity in the middle of the chest. It contains the internal organs in the chest except for the lungs. These organs include the heart, **bronchial tubes, esophagus,** *aorta,* and **trachea.** Finding a **mediastinal** mass on a chest x-ray may indicate the presence of a tumor in the area between the lungs.

> *Aorta: largest artery in the body*

4. MRI Report of the Cervical Spine

Patient has a clinical history of shoulder pain. Findings at C2-3 are normal. Findings at C3-4 indicate a small central **disk (disc)** *herniation.* C4-5 is normal. Findings at C5-6 show some bony outgrowths called *osteophytes* and slight narrowing of the **spinal cavity.**

> *Herniation: bulging or protrusion of an organ or structure*
> *Osteophytes: bony outgrowths*

Suffixes

This chapter presents suffixes and terms that illustrate the use of those suffixes. Some suffixes have been introduced previously (Chapters 1 and 2), whereas others are new. I begin teaching the chapter with Section III, Suffixes and Terminology, and explain each of the terms on the lists of Diagnostic and Procedural Suffixes. Included below are additional terms, which use the suffixes on the list. The suffix in each term is underlined.

Additional Suffixes and Terminology

Diagnostic Suffixes

cirrhosis	Literally means *abnormal condition* of yellow-orange, from the Greek *kirrhos*. The French physician Laennec named this disorder of the liver because he was impressed with the abnormal color of the scarred livers of alcoholics.
leukocytosis	*Abnormal condition* of white blood cells (slight increase in numbers).
scoliosis	*Abnormal condition* of the spine (lateral curvature). This term comes from the Greek *skoliosis,* meaning "a bending or curvature."
splenomegaly	*Enlargement* of the spleen.
melanoma	*Tumor* of melanocytes (pigmented, melanin-containing cells in the skin). This is a malignant tumor. Other malignant tumors that do not have CARCINOMA or SARCOMA in their names are:

Ewing tumor	tumor of bone (also called Ewing sarcoma)
hepatoma	tumor of the liver
Hodgkin disease	tumor of lymph nodes
hypernephroma	tumor of the kidney (also called renal cell carcinoma)
lymphoma	tumor of lymph nodes
multiple myeloma	tumor of bone marrow
Wilms tumor	tumor of the kidney (in children)

retinopathy	*Disease* of the retina of the eye. This condition is often a manifestation of diabetes mellitus, marked by dilation of retinal veins and arteries or the formation of new blood vessels that may eventually rupture and cause hemorrhage into the eye (vitreous humor).

osteo<u>pathy</u>	*Disease* of bones. More commonly, this term refers to a system of therapy involving manipulation of the skeletal system. It is founded on the theory that the body is capable of producing its own remedies against disease when its structure is normal and it has proper nutrition and a favorable environment.
leuko<u>rrhea</u>	White discharge (from the vagina).
pyo<u>rrhea</u>	Flow of pus. Collection of purulent material from infected tooth sockets, related to inflammation and disease of gums.
sebo<u>rrhea</u>	Excessive discharge of sebum (oil) from the skin, forming greasy scales or plugs on the body.
steato<u>rrhea</u>	Discharge of fat in the feces.
multiple <u>sclerosis</u>	*Hardening* of nerve fibers (axons of nerve cells). Scar tissue forms on nerve cells in scattered places in the brain and spinal cord. It causes weakness in muscles, often leading to loss of muscle coordination.
oto<u>sclerosis</u>	Abnormal formation *(hardening)* of new bone around a structure (oval window) in the inner ear. This prevents the stapes (middle ear bone) from moving and results in loss of hearing.
albumin<u>uria</u>	Protein (albumin) in the *urine* (abnormal condition).
glycos<u>uria</u>	Sugar in the *urine* (abnormal condition).
py<u>uria</u>	Pus in the *urine* (abnormal condition).

Procedural Suffixes

endarte<u>rectomy</u>	*Removal* of the inner lining of an artery (to remove plaque).
vit<u>rectomy</u>	*Removal* of the vitreous humor (performed as treatment for diabetic retinopathy).
abdomino<u>centesis</u>	Surgical puncture to remove fluid from the abdomen. Also called a paracentesis.
acetabulo<u>plasty</u>	Surgical repair of the acetabulum (hip socket).
arthro<u>plasty</u>	Surgical repair of a joint.
blepharo<u>plasty</u>	Surgical repair of the eyelid.
tympano<u>plasty</u>	Surgical repair of the eardrum.
valvulo<u>plasty</u>	Surgical repair of a valve within the heart.
ileo<u>stomy</u>	*Opening* of the ileum to the outside of the body. This may be temporary or permanent. When it is done in conjunction with removal of the colon and anus, it is always permanent.
hydro<u>therapy</u>	Treatment with water; whirlpool baths.
psycho<u>therapy</u>	Treatment of the mind.
choledocholitho<u>tomy</u>	*Incision* of the common bile duct (CHOLEDOCH/O) to remove a stone (LITH).
episio<u>tomy</u>	*Incision* of the perineum (area between the anus and the vagina). This is done to facilitate delivery of the infant.
myringo<u>tomy</u>	*Incision* of the eardrum to provide drainage of purulent collections in the middle ear.
nephrolitho<u>tomy</u>	*Incision* of the kidney to remove a stone.

Chapter 3   Multiple Choice Quiz

1. -osis means:
   - A. inflammation
   - B. tumor
   - C. pain
   - D. abnormal condition
   - E. visual examination

2. Blood infection:
   - A. anemia
   - B. septicemia
   - C. meningitis
   - D. hematoma
   - E. hemorrhage

3. Ear pain:
   - A. colitis
   - B. rhinalgia
   - C. myalgia
   - D. arthritis
   - E. otalgia

4. A condition in which blood is held back from an organ:
   - A. ischemia
   - B. uremia
   - C. hematuria
   - D. leukemia
   - E. menorrhea

5. A benign tumor of muscle is a(an):
   - A. adenoma
   - B. adenocarcinoma
   - C. myoma
   - D. myosarcoma
   - E. myocardial infarction

6. Renal failure leads to this abnormal blood condition:
   - A. vasculitis
   - B. cystitis
   - C. menorrhagia
   - D. thrombosis
   - E. uremia

7. Enlargement of the liver:
   - A. hepatomegaly
   - B. nephritis
   - C. hepatitis
   - D. cardiomegaly
   - E. nephromegaly

8. Inflammation of the membranes around the brain and spinal cord:
   - A. neuralgia
   - B. encephalitis
   - C. pleuritis
   - D. meningitis
   - E. encephalopathy

9. The large intestine is called the:
   - A. larynx
   - B. pharynx
   - C. esophagus
   - D. trachea
   - E. colon

10. Disease of heart muscle:
    - A. myosarcoma
    - B. arthropathy
    - C. cardiomyopathy
    - D. nephropathy
    - E. neuritis

11. A cancerous tumor of glandular (epithelial) cells is called:
    - A. leukemia
    - B. hematuria
    - C. adenoma
    - D. adenocarcinoma
    - E. sarcoma

12. Discharge of blood during the menstrual period is called:
    - A. hemorrhage
    - B. menorrhea
    - C. rhinorrhea
    - D. anemia
    - E. hematuria

13. A suffix meaning a condition of hardening is:
    - A. -centesis
    - B. -arteri/o
    - C. -pathy
    - D. -plasty
    - E. -sclerosis

14. Pertaining to the groin:
    - A. inguinal
    - B. renal
    - C. pelvic
    - D. peritoneal
    - E. lateral

15. Condition of blood in the urine:
    A. uremia
    B. menorrhagia
    C. hematuria
    D. hematology
    E. ischemia

16. A myocardial infarction is a(an):
    A. stroke
    B. heart attack
    C. disease of the brain
    D. enlargement of the liver
    E. inflammation of a joint

17. A condition that lasts for a long time is called:
    A. acute
    B. septic
    C. lateral
    D. coccygeal
    E. chronic

18. A suffix that means resection is:
    A. -tomy
    B. -plasty
    C. -ectomy
    D. -stomy
    E. -therapy

19. Surgical puncture to remove fluid from the sac around the fetus is:
    A. arthrocentesis
    B. arteriosclerosis
    C. hysterectomy
    D. laparotomy
    E. amniocentesis

20. Removal of a fallopian tube:
    A. hysterotomy
    B. colectomy
    C. thoracocentesis
    D. salpingectomy
    E. oophorectomy

21. X-ray record of the spinal cord:
    A. mammogram
    B. myelogram
    C. mammography
    D. electromyogram
    E. arthrogram

22. Removal of pharyngeal lymph tissue:
    A. tonsillectomy
    B. mastectomy
    C. nephrectomy
    D. neurotomy
    E. tracheotomy

23. Surgical repair of breast tissue:
    A. hysterosalpingectomy
    B. mastitis
    C. mammography
    D. mammoplasty
    E. rhinoplasty

24. Separation of waste (urea) from the blood by filtration through a machine:
    A. electroencephalography
    B. arthrocentesis
    C. peritoneal dialysis
    D. abdominocentesis
    E. hemodialysis

25. Combining form for blood vessel:
    A. angi/o
    B. erythr/o
    C. hem/o
    D. leuk/o
    E. arthr/o

26. Creation of a new opening from the windpipe to the outside of the body:
    A. laryngotomy
    B. pharyngotomy
    C. laparoscopy
    D. tracheostomy
    E. colostomy

27. Treatment using drugs:
    A. chemotherapy
    B. radiotherapy
    C. hemodialysis
    D. angioplasty
    E. myelography

28. Incision of the abdomen:
    A. arthrotomy
    B. abdominoplasty
    C. cholecystectomy
    D. laparotomy
    E. craniotomy

Chapter 3   Spelling and Comprehension Quiz

I. Spelling

1. _____   11. _____

2. _____   12. _____

3. _____   13. _____

4. _____   14. _____

5. _____   15. _____

6. _____   16. _____

7. _____   17. _____

8. _____   18. _____

9. _____   19. _____

10. _____   20. _____

II. Comprehension: Match the terms listed above with their meanings below.

_____ enlargement of the liver

_____ inflammation of the urinary bladder

_____ menstrual flow

_____ ear pain

_____ holding back blood from an area of the body

_____ hardening of the arteries

_____ malignant tumor of a gland

_____ blood in the urine

_____ disease of heart muscle

_____ nerve pain

_____ resection of a fallopian tube

_____ high levels of urea in the blood

_____ inflammation of membranes surrounding the brain

_____ infection in the blood

_____ surgical puncture to remove fluid from the chest

_____ abnormal condition of death of cells

_____ malignant tumor of muscle

_____ surgical puncture to remove fluid from the sac surrounding the embryo

_____ inflammation of the large intestine

_____ bursting forth of blood

III. Match the combining form in Column I with its meaning in Column II.

Column I		Column II
1. hyster/o	_____	A. armpit
2. ren/o	_____	B. vein
3. oophor/o	_____	C. breast
4. axill/o	_____	D. bronchial tube
5. inguin/o	_____	E. kidney
6. vascul/o	_____	F. joint
7. mast/o	_____	G. spinal cord and bone marrow
8. pneumon/o	_____	H. blood vessel
9. myel/o	_____	I. uterus
10. arthr/o	_____	J. lung
11. bronch/o	_____	K. groin
12. phleb/o	_____	L. ovary

Chapter 3   Review Quiz

I. Give meanings for the following suffixes:

1. -megaly _____
2. -sclerosis _____
3. -centesis _____
4. -stomy _____
5. -uria _____
6. -rrhagia _____
7. -pathy _____
8. -lysis _____

9. -therapy _____
10. -plasty _____
11. -gram _____
12. -tomy _____
13. -ary _____
14. -osis _____
15. -eal _____

II. Give meanings for the following combining forms:

1. angi/o _____
2. aden/o _____
3. arteri/o _____
4. amni/o _____
5. ren/o _____
6. sarc/o _____
7. my/o _____
8. oste/o _____
9. chron/o _____
10. inguin/o _____
11. mamm/o _____
12. nephr/o _____
13. men/o _____

14. encephal/o _____
15. carcin/o _____
16. cry/o _____
17. chem/o _____
18. isch/o _____
19. necr/o _____
20. radi/o _____
21. septic/o _____
22. vascul/o _____
23. thorac/o _____
24. ur/o _____
25. ather/o _____

44

III. Give combining forms for the following parts of the body:

1. gallbladder _____
2. armpit _____
3. urinary bladder _____
4. ovary _____
5. ear _____
6. nose _____
7. fallopian tube _____
8. liver _____
9. uterus _____
10. colon _____
11. heart _____
12. joint _____
13. vein _____

14. bone marrow _____
15. spinal cord _____
16. membranes surrounding the brain and spinal cord _____
17. voice box _____
18. blood _____
19. hip bones _____
20. skull _____
21. windpipe _____
22. tonsils _____
23. membrane surrounding the abdomen _____
24. esophagus _____
25. tubes from the trachea to the lungs _____

Chapter 3 Crossword Puzzle Quiz

Across

5. flow or discharge from the nose
8. suffix meaning *pain*
9. new opening into the colon from the outside of the body
10. pain of a muscle
11. suffix meaning *disease*
12. x-ray record of the spinal cord
14. suffix meaning *new opening*
15. blood in the urine

Down

1. pain of a joint
2. excision or removal of tonsils
3. cancerous tumor
4. suffix meaning *treatment*
6. suffix meaning *inflammation*
7. suffix meaning *hardening*
13. suffix meaning *tumor* or *mass*

Chapter 3   Answers

Multiple Choice

1. D	15. C
2. B	16. B
3. E	17. E
4. A	18. C
5. C	19. E
6. E	20. D
7. A	21. B
8. D	22. A
9. E	23. D
10. C	24. E
11. D	25. A
12. B	26. D
13. E	27. A
14. A	28. D

Spelling and Comprehension Quiz

I. Spelling

1. adenocarcinoma
2. amniocentesis
3. arteriosclerosis
4. cardiomyopathy
5. colitis
6. cystitis
7. hematuria
8. hemorrhage
9. hepatomegaly
10. ischemia
11. meningitis
12. menorrhea
13. myosarcoma
14. necrosis
15. neuralgia
16. otalgia
17. salpingectomy
18. septicemia
19. thoracentesis
20. uremia

II. Comprehension

9   enlargement of the liver
6   inflammation of the urinary bladder
12   menstrual flow
16   ear pain
10   holding back blood from an area of the body
3   hardening of arteries
1   malignant tumor of a gland
7   blood in the urine
4   disease of heart muscle
15   nerve pain
17   resection of a fallopian tube
20   high levels of urea in the blood
11   inflammation of membranes surrounding the brain
18   infection in the blood
19   surgical puncture to remove fluid from the chest
14   abnormal condition of death of cells
13   malignant tumor of muscle
2   surgical puncture to remove fluid from the sac surrounding the embryo
5   inflammation of the large intestine
8   bursting forth of blood

III. Matching

1. I
2. E
3. L
4. A
5. K
6. H
7. C
8. J
9. G
10. F
11. D
12. B

Review Quiz

I.
1. enlargement
2. hardening
3. surgical procedure to remove fluid
4. new opening (to form a mouth)
5. urination; condition of urine
6. bursting forth (of blood)
7. disease, condition
8. separation, destruction, breakdown
9. treatment
10. surgical repair
11. record
12. incision
13. pertaining to
14. abnormal condition
15. pertaining to

II.
1. blood vessel
2. gland
3. artery
4. amnion
5. kidney
6. flesh
7. muscle
8. bone
9. time
10. groin
11. breast
12. kidney
13. menstruation
14. brain
15. cancerous
16. cold
17. drug, chemical
18. to hold back
19. death
20. x-rays
21. pertaining to infection
22. blood vessel
23. chest
24. urine; urinary tract
25. plaque, collection of fatty material

III.
1. cholecyst/o
2. axill/o
3. cyst/o
4. oophor/o
5. ot/o
6. rhin/o
7. salping/o
8. hepat/o
9. hyster/o
10. col/o
11. cardi/o
12. arthr/o
13. phleb/o
14. myel/o
15. myel/o
16. mening/o
17. laryng/o
18. hemat/o
19. pelv/o
20. crani/o
21. trache/o
22. tonsill/o
23. peritone/o
24. esophag/o
25. bronch/o

Crossword Puzzle Quiz

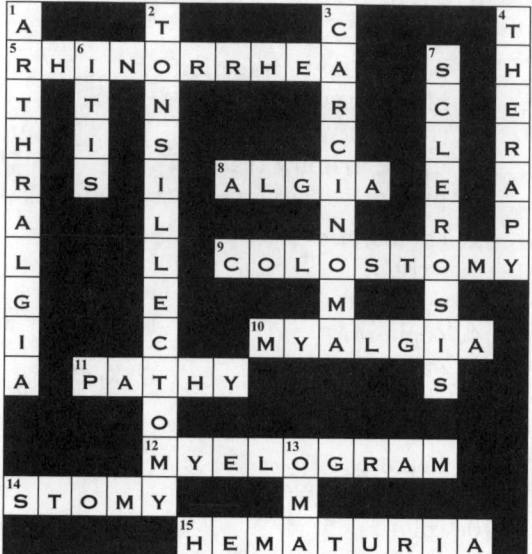

Dictation Sentences

Medical terms that are in **bold** are found in the chapter. Italicized terms may be new to students. Their definitions follow the paragraph.

1. Operative Report: Bronchoscopy

Findings: **Bronchoscopy** through the *endotracheal tube* showed a normal *distal* **trachea.** The *carina* and the left and right **tracheobronchial** systems were entirely normal. All of the segmental **bronchi** were widely *patent* inside the chest.

> *Carina: part of the trachea that branches to form the bronchial tubes*
> *Distal: farthest from the beginning of an organ or tube*
> *Endotracheal tube: an airway tube inserted through the mouth into the windpipe*
> *Patent: open*

2. Myocardial Infarction

A **myocardial infarction,** or heart attack, is an area of dead tissue in heart muscle. It can occur when **atherosclerosis** blocks a *coronary* artery and *occludes* it. **Ischemia** follows as blood fails to reach the heart muscle. Because the blood, carrying necessary food and oxygen, never reaches the heart muscle, **necrosis** or **infarction** occurs.

> *Coronary: pertaining to the heart*
> *Occluded: closed off*

3. Angiography and Angioplasty

Angiography visualizes the coronary arteries. X-ray images show **arteriosclerosis** after *contrast* is injected into a blood vessel. **Angioplasty** may then be performed to open clogged arteries. Using a *catheter* containing a balloon and a *stent,* angioplasty keeps a clogged artery open and is an alternative to *coronary bypass surgery (CABG).*

> *Catheter: a tube for injecting or withdrawing fluid*
> *Contrast: material injected to visualize parts of the body on an x-ray*
> *Coronary bypass surgery (CABG): open heart surgery using veins and arteries in place of*
>   *clogged coronary arteries (coronary artery bypass graft)*
> *Stent: slotted tube*

4. Electroencephalogram Report

Interpretation: Abnormal EEG, characterized by *bihemispheric* slowing with some *focality* noted in the right *parietal* area. This may be explained by *diffuse metabolic* disturbance in the right *hemisphere,* as would be seen in a mass lesion or from a **cerebrovascular accident.** No evidence of any *epileptic* activity is seen.

> *Bihemispheric: pertaining to both (bi- = two) hemispheres or halves of the brain*
> *Diffuse: becoming widely spread*
> *Epileptic: pertaining to epilepsy or seizure disorder in the brain*
> *Focality: localized area of abnormal nerve cell discharges*
> *Hemisphere: half of the brain*
> *Metabolic: pertaining to metabolism (chemical activity of cells)*
> *Parietal: pertaining to the side and middle part of the cerebrum*

Chapter 4

Prefixes

This chapter reviews prefixes that have been used in previous chapters and adds new prefixes as well. The following additional terms may be helpful in providing further examples of prefixes explained in the chapter. Prefixes are underlined in each term.

Additional Prefixes and Terminology

<u>an</u>esthesia	*No* sensation. The loss of perception of pain or touch in a part of the body; or the procedures whereby a patient has been incapable of sensation by inducing a state of total unconsciousness or by blocking the nerve pathway to a part of the body. From the Greek *aisthesis*, meaning "feeling or sensation."
<u>an</u>orexia	*No* (lack of) appetite. From the Greek *orexis*, meaning "appetite."
<u>a</u>taxia	*Without* coordination. From the Greek *taxis*, meaning "order or arrangement." The term means a lack of motor coordination, particularly that of gait (manner of walking), and is caused by damage to the cerebellum (lower, posterior part of the brain).
<u>ab</u>duct	To draw or lead *away* from the body. From the Latin *abducere*, meaning "to lead away." An abductor muscle pulls the limb away from the trunk of the body.
<u>ad</u>duct	To draw or lead *toward* the body. An adductor muscle draws a limb toward the body.
<u>anti</u>dote	An agent administered to work *against* a poison. From the Greek *anti*, meaning "against," and *dotos*, meaning "what is given."
<u>anti</u>sepsis	*Against* infection. A treatment that makes an object free of infection. From the Greek *anti* and *sepsis*, meaning "putrefaction."
<u>con</u>junctiva	The transparent membrane covering the eyeball. From the Latin meaning "connecting or joining together." The conjunctiva *connects* the globe of the eye with the lid.
<u>dys</u>pareunia	*Painful* sexual intercourse. From the Greek *pareunos*, meaning "lying beside."
<u>dys</u>pepsia	*Difficult* digestion. From the Greek *pepsis*, meaning "digestion."
<u>dys</u>trophy	*Abnormal* growth and development; from the Greek *trophe*, meaning "nourishment."
<u>endo</u>metrium	*Inner* lining of the uterus. From the Greek *metra*, meaning "uterus."

epiglottis	The flap of cartilage *above* the entrance to the trachea. The structure was once thought of as an appendage of the tongue. From the Greek *glossa,* meaning "tongue."
exophthalmos	Protruding ("out") eyeball. Exophthalmic goiter is a condition of enlargement of the thyroid gland associated with bulging of the white of the eye (sclera).
malaise	A vague feeling of bodily discomfort. From the French *mal,* meaning "bad" or "ill," and *aise,* meaning "ease."
prodrome	Early stage of an illness; that which "runs *before.*" From the Greek *dromos,* meaning "running."
trimester	The equally divided early, middle, and late stages of pregnancy. The term means a period of *three* months, from *mestris,* meaning "monthly."
ultraviolet	Of a wavelength above and *beyond* that of visible violet light.

Chapter 4   Multiple Choice Quiz

1. Not able to breathe:
   - A. atrophy
   - B. tachypnea
   - C. dysplasia
   - D. dyspnea
   - E. apnea

2. Before birth:
   - A. antigen
   - B. antepartum
   - C. postpartum
   - D. postnatal
   - E. neonatal

3. Deficiency in red blood cells or of the hemoglobin within the red cells:
   - A. antigen
   - B. antepartum
   - C. postpartum
   - D. postnatal
   - E. nesonatal

4. Excessive (more than normal) development:
   - A. hypoplasia
   - B. dysplasia
   - C. atrophy
   - D. hypertrophy
   - E. neoplastic

5. A return of symptoms of illness:
   - A. remission
   - B. resection
   - C. prolapse
   - D. prosthesis
   - E. relapse

6. Difficult, painful urination:
   - A. urinalysis
   - B. dysuria
   - C. polyuria
   - D. hematuria
   - E. uremia

7. A protein made by white blood cells and capable of destroying bacteria and viruses:
   - A. antibody
   - B. antibiotic
   - C. antigen
   - D. hemoglobin
   - E. leukocyte

8. An irregularity that occurs at birth:
   - A. intrauterine
   - B. neonatal
   - C. benign
   - D. congenital anomaly
   - E. ectopic pregnancy

9. Slow heartbeat:
   - A. bradycardia
   - B. tachypnea
   - C. cardiomegaly
   - D. myocardial infarction
   - E. tachycardia

10. An artificial part:
    - A. metacarpal
    - B. epidermis
    - C. prosthesis
    - D. anomaly
    - E. intervertebral disk

11. Pertaining to under the shoulder bone:
    - A. subcostal
    - B. hypodermic
    - C. subdural
    - D. epidural
    - E. subscapular

12. Pertaining to both (two) sides:
    - A. unilateral
    - B. tricuspid
    - C. intravenous
    - D. sagittal
    - E. bilateral

13. Process of recording sound waves to make an image of organs in the body:
    - A. CT scan
    - B. ultrasonography
    - C. MRI
    - D. endoscopy
    - E. dialysis

14. Endocrine glands that are near (above) each kidney:
    - A. adrenal
    - B. prostate
    - C. subcostal
    - D. parathyroid
    - E. transurethral

15. The spread of a cancerous tumor to another organ away from the original location:
    A. subcutaneous
    B. carcinoma
    C. neoplastic
    D. metastasis
    E. malignant

16. Two prefixes that mean "beyond":
    A. tachy- and brady-
    B. pro- and pre-
    C. dys- and mal-
    D. re- and retro-
    E. ultra- and meta-

17. A word that means "complete separation" and is the process of separating wastes from the blood:
    A. dialysis
    B. diarrhea
    C. urinalysis
    D. syndrome
    E. subcutaneous

18. A membrane that surrounds bone:
    A. pericardium
    B. peritoneum
    C. epidermis
    D. subcostal
    E. periosteum

19. A prefix that has the same meaning as "ante" is:
    A. a-, an-
    B. anti-
    C. pro-
    D. ad-
    E. pan-

20. Poly- has a similar meaning with:
    A. re-
    B. dys-
    C. syn-
    D. hyper-
    E. hypo-

21. A group of symptoms that occur together is called a(an):
    A. analysis
    B. syndrome
    C. dialysis
    D. prognosis
    E. remission

22. A prefix that means "near, along the side of" is:
    A. neo-
    B. pro-
    C. peri-
    D. para-
    E. dia-

23. An abnormal collection of blood above the membrane covering the brain:
    A. subdural hematoma
    B. cerebral hemorrhage
    C. thrombosis
    D. epidural hematoma
    E. subdural hemorrhage

24. Two prefixes that mean "within":
    A. ante- and pro-
    B. endo- and intra-
    C. hypo- and sub-
    D. syn- and con-
    E. extra- and ec-

25. If an organ slides or falls forward, the condition is called:
    A. neoplasm
    B. relapse
    C. remission
    D. prolapse
    E. dysmenorrhea

Chapter 4 Spelling and Comprehension Quiz

I. Spelling

1. _____   11. _____

2. _____   12. _____

3. _____   13. _____

4. _____   14. _____

5. _____   15. _____

6. _____   16. _____

7. _____   17. _____

8. _____   18. _____

9. _____   19. _____

10. _____   20. _____

II. Comprehension: Match the terms listed above with their meanings below.

_____ within the uterus

_____ difficult breathing

_____ pertaining to a newborn

_____ painful urination

_____ after birth

_____ spread of a cancerous (malignant tumor)

_____ low blood sugar

_____ collection of blood above a meningeal layer

_____ excessive development

_____ discharge of fluid from the rectum

_____ slow heartbeat

_____ loss of movement due to nerve damage

_____ between a backbone

_____ embryo is not in the proper location

_____ pertaining to one side

_____ abnormal growth or development

_____ harmless, noncancerous

_____ falling down; drooping of a part of the body

_____ artificial part attached to the body

_____ cancerous; harmful

III. Match the term in Column I with its meaning in Column II.

Column I		Column II
1. metacarpal	_____	A. behind the abdominal cavity
2. remission	_____	B. below the shoulder blade
3. subscapular	_____	C. membrane surrounding a bone
4. perianal	_____	D. abnormality present at birth
5. relapse	_____	E. foreign body; bacteria, virus
6. subcostal	_____	F. symptoms of disease return
7. periosteum	_____	G. pertaining to surrounding the anus
8. retroperitoneal	_____	H. symptoms of disease disappear
9. congenital anomaly	_____	I. under the ribs
10. antigen	_____	J. hand bone

Review Quiz

I. Give meanings for the following prefixes:

1. ante- _____
2. anti- _____
3. epi- _____
4. ab- _____
5. ad- _____
6. hemi- _____
7. hyper- _____
8. inter- _____

9. intra- _____
10. post- _____
11. meta- _____
12. hypo- _____
13. para- _____
14. syn- _____
15. mal- _____

II. Give prefixes for the following English terms:

1. one _____
2. two _____
3. three _____
4. four _____

5. surrounding _____
6. new _____
7. fast _____
8. slow _____

III. Give meanings for the following suffixes:

1. -pnea _____
2. -tension _____
3. -uria _____
4. -dipsia _____
5. -gen _____
6. -emia _____
7. -lysis _____
8. -partum _____

9. -pathy _____
10. -rrhea _____
11. -stasis _____
12. -mortem _____
13. -plasm _____
14. -graphy _____
15. -tic _____

Chapter 4   Crossword Puzzle Quiz

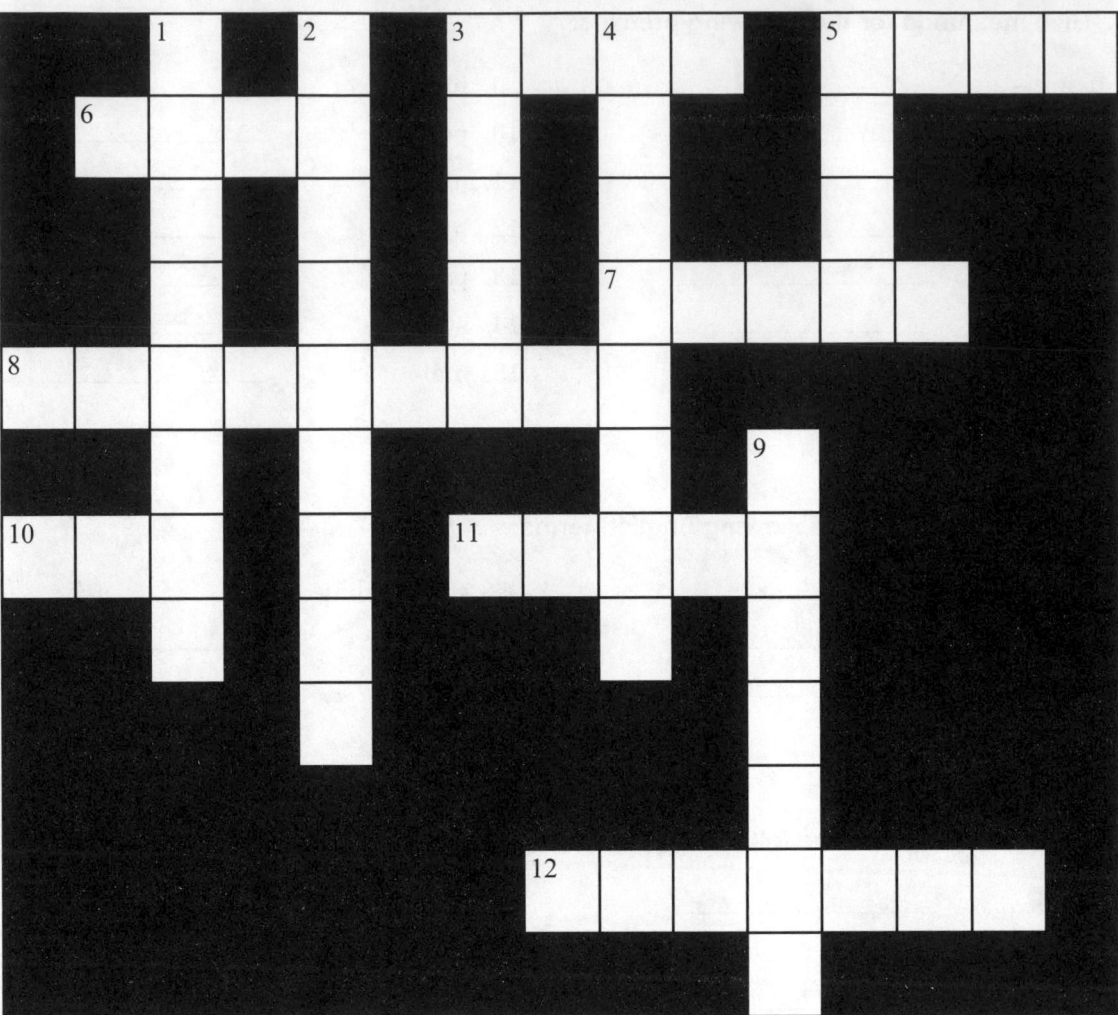

Across

3. prefix meaning *below* or *deficient*
5. prefix meaning *against*
6. prefix meaning *beyond*
7. prefix meaning *between*
8. slow discharge of urine
10. prefix meaning *up* or *apart*
11. prefix meaning *slow*
12. benign tumor of bone

Down

1. pertaining to new birth
2. rapid breathing
3. prefix meaning *above* or *excessive*
4. surrounding the anus
5. prefix meaning *before*
9. painful breathing

Chapter 4   Answers

Multiple Choice

1. E	14. A
2. B	15. D
3. C	16. E
4. D	17. A
5. E	18. E
6. B	19. C
7. A	20. D
8. D	21. B
9. A	22. D
10. C	23. D
11. E	24. B
12. E	25. D
13. B	

Spelling and Comprehension Quiz

I. Spelling

1. benign
2. bradycardia
3. diarrhea
4. dysplasia
5. dyspnea
6. dysuria
7. ectopic pregnancy
8. epidural hematoma
9. hypertrophy
10. hypoglycemia
11. intervertebral
12. intrauterine
13. malignant
14. metastasis
15. neonatal
16. paralysis
17. postpartum
18. prolapse
19. prosthesis
20. unilateral

II. Comprehension

12 within the uterus
5 difficult breathing
15 pertaining to a newborn
6 painful urination
17 after birth
14 spread of a cancerous (malignant) tumor
10 low blood sugar
8 collection of blood above a meningeal layer
9 excessive development
3 discharge of fluid from the rectum
2 slow heartbeat
16 loss of movement due to nerve damage
11 between a backbone
7 embryo is not in the proper location
20 pertaining to one side
4 abnormal growth or development
1 harmless, noncancerous
18 falling down; drooping of a part of the body
19 artificial part attached to the body
13 cancerous; harmful

III. Matching

1. J
2. H
3. B
4. G
5. F
6. I
7. C
8. A
9. D
10. E

Review Quiz

I. 1. before, forward
2. against
3. above, upon
4. away from
5. toward; near
6. half
7. excessive, above
8. between
9. within
10. after, behind
11. change; beyond
12. below, under
13. beside, near, along the side of
14. with, together
15. bad

II. 1. uni-
2. bi-
3. tri-
4. quadri-
5. peri-
6. neo-
7. tachy-
8. brady-

III. 1. breathing
2. pressure
3. urine condition
4. thirst
5. to produce
6. blood condition
7. loosening,
   breakdown, separation, destruction
8. birth
9. disease condition
10. flow, discharge
11. to stand, place, stop, control
12. death
13. formation
14. process of recording
15. pertaining to

Crossword Puzzle Quiz

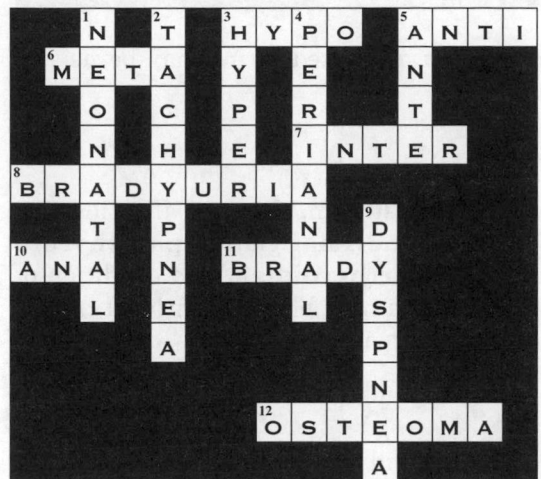

Dictation Sentences

Medical terms that are in **bold** are found in the chapter. Italicized terms may be new to students. Their definitions follow the paragraph.

1. Endocrine Glands

Endocrine glands secrete hormones through the bloodstream, directly affecting the function of organs. Examples of endocrine glands are the **adrenal** glands, **parathyroid** glands, thyroid gland, pituitary gland, and pancreas. **Hyperthyroidism** is a condition of excessive secretion of thyroid hormone. **Hyperglycemia** is a high blood sugar level caused by deficient secretion of the hormone insulin from the pancreas.

2. Malignant Tumors

There are two types of **malignant** tumors, **carcinomas** and **sarcomas.** Carcinomas are cancerous tumors arising from **epithelial** cells, which are lining cells in internal organs such as the lung, urinary bladder, gastrointestinal tract, and glands. Often, these cancerous tumors are called **adenocarcinomas. Sarcomas** arise from connective tissues, such as muscle, bone, cartilage, and fat. An example of a sarcoma is an *osteosarcoma*. The main characteristic of a **malignant neoplasm** is **metastasis.** If the tumor is treated with **resection,** chemotherapy, and/or radiotherapy, **remission** and cure are possible. If **relapse** occurs, the patient may require further treatment.

> *Osteosarcoma: malignant tumor of bone*

3. Congenital Anomaly

A **congenital anomaly** is a birth defect. Examples of **neonatal** abnormalities include Down **syndrome,** hip **dysplasia,** sickle cell **anemia,** heart defects, and *spina bifida,* which may involve **paralysis.** If the **congenital anomaly** arises from the genes in egg and sperm cells, it is *hereditary*. If it arises from the **antenatal intrauterine** environment, it is acquired.

> *Hereditary: a condition transmitted from parent to offspring via genes*
> *Spina bifida: a congenital defect of the spine in which there is a gap in the vertebrae that causes outward bulging of the spinal cord and/or meninges*

Medical Specialists
and Case Reports

This chapter describes the training process of physicians and gives the names of medical specialists. In addition, combining forms found in the names of medical specialists are reviewed and then used with suffixes to illustrate their meaning. Also included in the chapter are short case reports from medical specialties. The reports use medical terms studied in the text and include others to expand the student's vocabulary. All terms are defined in the *Glossary of Medical Terms*. Reading and deciphering these reports in class will convince students that they can now understand the medical language.

Two class activities are included here. Matching Exercises for Medical Specialists (A and B) (see pp. 64-65) test knowledge of medical specialists. Matching Exercises for the Case Reports (see pp. 67-71) review terms used in the individual reports in the text. Students read these reports aloud, and I ask questions to help them understand the meaning of terms. The boldfaced terms are defined in the *Glossary of Medical Terms,* so students can look up meanings easily. Answers to class activities follow each one.

64

Matching Exercises for Medical Specialists

A. Match the following specialists with their specialties listed below.

allergist   geriatrician
anesthesiologist   gynecologist
cardiologist   hematologist
cardiovascular surgeon   infectious disease specialist
colorectal surgeon   nephrologist
dermatologist   neurologist
endocrinologist   neurosurgeon
gastroenterologist

1. Treatment of kidney disease: _____

2. Treatment (with drugs) of heart disease: _____

3. Treatment of hypersensitivity reactions: _____

4. Surgery on the brain, spinal cord, and nerves: _____

5. Surgery on the large intestine (colon and rectum): _____

6. Treatment of skin disorders: _____

7. Treatment of blood disorders: _____

8. Diagnosis and treatment of nerve disorders: _____

9. Treatment of endocrine gland disorders: _____

10. Surgery on the female reproductive tract: _____

11. Treatment of diseases of old age: _____

12. Surgery on the heart and blood vessels: _____

13. Treatment of diseases caused by microorganisms: _____

14. Treatment of stomach and intestinal disorders: _____

15. Administration of agents for loss of sensation: _____

B. Match the following specialists with their specialties.

obstetrician	psychiatrist
oncologist	pulmonary specialist
ophthalmologist	radiation oncologist
orthopedist	radiologist
otolaryngologist	rheumatologist
pathologist	thoracic surgeon
pediatrician	urologist
physical medicine and rehabilitation specialist	

1. Surgery on the urinary tract: _____

2. Treatment of pregnant women; delivery of babies _____

3. Treatment of joint and muscle disorders: _____

4. Surgery on chest organs: _____

5. Drug treatment of malignant tumors: _____

6. Treatment of mental disorders: _____

7. Treatment to restore function after illness: _____

8. Treatment of disease with high-energy radiation: _____

9. Treatment of the ear, nose, and throat: _____

10. Surgical treatment of bones, muscles, and joints: _____

11. Treatment of lung disorders: _____

12. Diagnosis of disease by analysis of cells and tissues: _____

13. Examination of radiographs to determine a diagnosis: _____

14. Treatment of diseases of children: _____

15. Surgical and medical treatment of eye disorders: _____

Answers to Matching Exercises for Medical Specialists

A.

1. nephrologist
2. cardiologist
3. allergist
4. neurosurgeon
5. colorectal surgeon
6. dermatologist
7. hematologist
8. neurologist

9. endocrinologist
10. gynecologist
11. geriatrician
12. cardiovascular surgeon
13. infectious disease specialist
14. gastroenterologist
15. anesthesiologist

B.

1. urologist
2. obstetrician
3. rheumatologist
4. thoracic surgeon
5. oncologist
6. psychiatrist
7. physical medicine and rehabilitation specialist

8. radiation oncologist
9. otorhinolaryngologist
10. orthopedist
11. pulmonary specialist
12. pathologist
13. radiologist
14. pediatrician
15. ophthalmologist

Matching Exercises for the Case Reports

Cardiology: Match each term with its meaning.

angina   hypertension
antiarrhythmic   ischemia
anticoagulant   myocardial infarction
diuretic

1. High blood pressure: _____

2. A drug that causes the kidneys to
   allow more fluid to leave the body: _____

3. Area of dead tissue within heart muscle;
   heart attack: _____

4. Drug that prevents clotting: _____

5. Deficiency of blood flow to a part of the body: _____

6. Sharp pain in the chest resulting from
   decrease in blood supply to the heart muscle: _____

7. A drug that works against or prevents
   abnormal heart beats: _____

Gynecology: Match each term with its meaning.

anemic   menorrhagia
dysmenorrhea   pelvic
fibroids   sonogram
hysterectomy   ultrasound

1. Removal of the uterus: _____

2. Benign growths of muscle tissue in the uterus: _____

3. Pertaining to a condition of less than normal
   numbers of red blood cells or of hemoglobin
   inside the red cells: _____

4. Sound waves with greater frequency than
   can be heard by the human ear: _____

5. Excessive bleeding from the uterus during
   the time of menstruation: _____

6. A record of sound waves after they bounce
   off organs in the body: _____

7. Painful menstrual flow: _____

8. Pertaining to the hip region: _____

68

Oncology: Match each term with its meaning.

biopsy   lymphangiography
hepatic   mediastinal
Hodgkin disease   percutaneous
intra-abdominal   peritoneoscopy
lymphangiogram   platelet

1. Process of viewing the membrane
   that surrounds the abdomen: _____

2. Pertaining to the central section of
   the chest, between the lungs: _____

3. Pertaining to through the skin: _____

4. Malignant tumor of lymph nodes: _____

5. Cell in the blood that helps blood to clot: _____

6. Pertaining to the liver: _____

7. Process of viewing living tissue by
   microscopic examination: _____

8. Process of recording (by x-ray) lymph
   vessels after dye is injected into lymph
   tissue in the soft part of the foot: _____

9. Pertaining to within the abdomen: _____

10. Record (x-ray) of lymph vessels after
    dye is injected into lymph tissue in
    the soft part of the foot: _____

Urology: Match each term with its meaning.

calculus   intravenous pyelogram
cystoscopy   lithotripsy
dysuria   prognosis
hematuria   renal

1. Forecast of the probable outcome
   of an illness or treatment: _____

2. Process of crushing a stone in the
   urinary tract using ultrasonic vibrations: _____

3. Process of viewing the urinary bladder using an
   endoscope (instrument with a light source and lens): _____

4. Abnormal condition of blood in urine: _____

5. X-ray record of the kidney after dye
   is injected into a vein: _____

6. A stone: _____

7. Painful urination: _____

8. Pertaining to the kidney: _____

Gastroenterology: Match each term with its meaning.

abdominal   gastrectomy
anemic   gastroscopy
barium swallow   hematemesis
dyspepsia   ulcer

1. Pertaining to a condition marked by reduced numbers of red blood cells or the amount of hemoglobin within the red cells: _____

2. A sore or a defect in the surface of an organ, which is produced by the destruction of tissue: _____

3. Pertaining to the space below the chest, containing organs such as the stomach, intestines, liver, and gallbladder: _____

4. An x-ray image of the upper digestive tract after swallowing a barium solution: _____

5. Vomiting blood: _____

6. Condition of painful digestion: _____

7. Excision of the stomach: _____

8. Visual examination of the stomach with an endoscope: _____

Radiology: Match each term with its meaning.

anterior   lobe   pneumonia
infiltrate   mediastinal   posterior
lateral   pleural effusion   thoracic cavity

1. Located in the back of a structure or of the body: _____

2. Located in the front of a structure or of the body: _____

3. Abnormal condition of the lungs marked by inflammation and collection of material within the air sacs: _____

4. Pertaining to a side: _____

5. A part or region of an organ, especially of the brain, lungs, or glands: _____

6. Space above the abdomen containing the heart and lungs: _____

7. Material that accumulates in an organ; often describing solid material and fluid collection in the lung: _____

8. Pertaining to the space between the lungs in the chest: _____

9. Collection of fluid between the membranes around the lungs: _____

Orthopedics: Match each term with its meaning.

femur   intra-abdominal
fixation   pelvis
fracture   tibia

1. The thigh bone: _____

2. Pertaining to within the abdomen: _____

3. Breaking of a bone: _____

4. The larger of the two lower leg bones: _____

5. Holding, sewing, or fastening a part in
   a fixed position: _____

6. Bones in the region of the hip: _____

Nephrology: Match each term with its meaning.

antihypertensive   hypertension
chronic   hypotensive
hemodialysis   renal failure

1. Lasting over a long period of time: _____

2. Use of a kidney machine to filter blood
   to remove waste materials: _____

3. High blood pressure: _____

4. Pertaining to low blood pressure: _____

5. Pertaining to a drug that reduces high
   blood pressure: _____

6. Stoppage of kidney function: _____

Endocrinology: Match each term with its meaning.

diabetes mellitus   polydipsia
insulin   polyuria

1. Excessive thirst: _____

2. Excessive urination: _____

3. Hormone produced by the pancreas: _____

4. Abnormal condition marked by deficient
   hormone in the blood; sugar cannot leave
   the blood to enter body cells: _____

Neurology: Match each term with its meaning.

acute   migraine
aura   nausea
cephalgia   unilateral
dilation   vasoconstrictor
frontal

1. Sharp, sudden, intense for a short period of time: _____

2. A drug that narrows blood vessels, especially
   small arteries: _____

3. Sensation that appears before more
   definite signs of illness: _____

4. Pain within the head (headache): _____

5. Pertaining to the anterior part: _____

6. Pertaining to one side: _____

7. Widening: _____

8. Unpleasant sensation in the upper
   abdomen, often leading to vomiting: _____

9. Particular attacks of head pain, usually caused
   by changes in blood vessel size and accompanied
   by nausea, vomiting, and sensitivity to light: _____

Answers to Matching Exercises for the Case Reports

Cardiology

1. hypertension
2. diuretic
3. myocardial infarction
4. anticoagulant
5. ischemia
6. angina
7. antiarrhythmic

Gynecology

1. hysterectomy
2. fibroids
3. anemic
4. ultrasound
5. menorrhagia
6. sonogram
7. dysmenorrhea
8. pelvic

Oncology

1. peritoneoscopy
2. mediastinum
3. percutaneous
4. Hodgkin disease
5. platelet
6. hepatic
7. biopsy
8. lymphangiography
9. intra-abdominal
10. lymphangiogram

Urology

1. prognosis
2. lithotripsy
3. cystoscopy
4. hematuria
5. intravenous pyelogram
6. calculus
7. dysuria
8. renal

Gastroenterology

1. anemic
2. ulcer
3. abdominal
4. barium swallow
5. hematemesis
6. dyspepsia
7. gastrectomy
8. gastroscopy

Radiology

1. posterior
2. anterior
3. pneumonia
4. lateral
5. lobe
6. thoracic cavity
7. infiltrate
8. mediastinum
9. pleural effusion

Orthopedics

1. femur
2. intra-abdominal
3. fracture
4. tibia
5. fixation
6. pelvis

Nephrology

1. chronic
2. hemodialysis
3. hypertension
4. hypotension
5. antihypertensive
6. renal failure

Endocrinology

1. polydipsia
2. polyuria
3. insulin
4. diabetes mellitus

Neurology

1. acute
2. vasoconstrictor
3. aura
4. cephalgia
5. frontal
6. unilateral
7. dilation
8. nausea
9. migrane

Chapter 5 Multiple Choice Quiz

1. A specialist in treating glandular disorders is a(an):
   A. gastroenterologist
   B. rheumatologist
   C. endocrinologist
   D. hematologist
   E. otolaryngologist

2. A doctor trained to treat eye disorders is a(an):
   A. oncologist
   B. optician
   C. optometrist
   D. orthopedist
   E. ophthalmologist

3. A surgeon specializing in disorders of the male reproductive system and urinary tract in males and females:
   A. nephrologist
   B. urologist
   C. gynecologist
   D. neurosurgeon
   E. colorectal surgeon

4. A doctor who treats lung disorders:
   A. cardiologist
   B. pathologist
   C. internist
   D. pulmonary specialist
   E. infectious disease specialist

5. A doctor who administers agents that cause loss of sensation during surgery:
   A. allergist
   B. cardiovascular surgeon
   C. oncologist
   D. neurologist
   E. anesthesiologist

6. A doctor specializing in treatment of disease using high-energy radiation:
   A. geriatrician
   B. pathologist
   C. radiologist
   D. radiation oncologist
   E. dermatologist

7. Internal medicine is a specialty concerned with:
   A. diagnosis of disease using x-rays
   B. care of patients who require sudden and immediate action
   C. diagnosis and treatment of children's disorders
   D. diagnosis and treatment of disorders of the mind
   E. diagnosis of disease and treatment with drugs

8. Clinical means:
   A. pertaining to time
   B. pertaining to the lung
   C. pertaining to patient care
   D. pertaining to skin disorders
   E. pertaining to laboratory research

9. A doctor who specializes in operating on the chest:
   A. thoracic surgeon
   B. colorectal surgeon
   C. otolaryngologist
   D. orthopedist
   E. oncologist

10. Which doctor specializes in treating older patients?
    A. family medicine specialist
    B. geriatrician
    C. rheumatologist
    D. pediatrician
    E. obstetrician

11. A disorder that is unexpectedly caused by treatment that is prescribed by a doctor is:
    A. neuralgic
    B. neurogenic
    C. oncogenic
    D. carcinogenic
    E. iatrogenic

12. An opening from the kidney to the outside of the body is a:
    A. thoracotomy
    B. tracheostomy
    C. laparotomy
    D. colostomy
    E. nephrostomy

13. Enlargement of the heart:
    A. hepatomegaly
    B. hematoma
    C. gastromegaly
    D. adenoma
    E. cardiomegaly

14. Instrument to view the eye:
    A. otoscopy
    B. otoscope
    C. ophthalmoscope
    D. laparoscope
    E. ophthalmoscopy

15. Discharge of fluid from the nose:
    A. rhinotomy
    B. rhinorrhea
    C. menorrhea
    D. dysmenorrhea
    E. rhinitis

16. A medical doctor who specializes in treating bone disorders is a(an):
    A. pathologist
    B. oncologist
    C. physical medicine and rehabilitation specialist
    D. orthopedist
    E. rheumatologist

17. Inflammation of the large intestine:
    A. enteritis
    B. colitis
    C. nephritis
    D. otitis
    E. hepatitis

18. Doctor who specializes in treatment of blood disorders:
    A. hematologist
    B. psychiatrist
    C. thoracic surgeon
    D. dermatologist
    E. cardiologist

19. Which term is *not* spelled correctly?
    A. laryngeal
    B. pulmonery
    C. vasculitis
    D. neuralgia
    E. gastroenterology

20. In which term is the pronunciation accent *incorrectly* placed?
    A. en-do-krin-OL-o-je
    B. ra-de-o-THER-ah-pe
    C. ko-LOS-to-me
    D. GAS-tros-ko-pe
    E. he-mah-TO-mah

Chapter 5   Spelling and Comprehension Quiz

I. Spelling

1. _____

2. _____

3. _____

4. _____

5. _____

6. _____

7. _____

8. _____

9. _____

10. _____

11. _____

12. _____

13. _____

14. _____

15. _____

16. _____

17. _____

18. _____

19. _____

20. _____

II. Comprehension: Match the terms listed above with their meanings below.

_____ new opening of the colon to the outside of the body

_____ study of administration of agents for loss of sensation

_____ inflammation of the voice box

_____ pain of nerves

_____ inflammation of the ear

_____ pertaining to an adverse condition produced by a treatment or physician

_____ inflammation of blood vessels

_____ physician who treats the mind and mental illness

_____ physician who treats disorders of the digestive system

_____ hernia of the rectum

_____ pertaining to producing a tumor

_____ incision of the chest

_____ physician who studies disease (reading biopsies and performing autopsies)

_____ process of visual examination of the stomach

_____ new opening of the kidney to the outside of the body

_____ discharge of fluid (mucus) from the nose

_____ treatment of pregnant women and delivery of babies

_____ physician who treats diseases of children

_____ physician who treats diseases of old age

_____ physician who treats disorders of the eye

III. Matching: Match the physician in Column I with the condition treated or procedure performed in Column II.

Column I

1. thoracic surgeon _____
2. otolaryngologist _____
3. cardiologist _____
4. neurosurgeon _____
5. orthopedist _____
6. hematologist _____
7. endocrinologist _____
8. urologist _____
9. oncologist _____
10. gynecologist _____

Column II

A. Hyperthyroidism
B. Cystitis
C. Vocal cord polyps
D. Cervical dysplasia
E. Pneumonectomy
F. Arthroscopy
G. Arrhythmia
H. Drug treatment of breast cancer
I. Sickle cell anemia
J. Resection of a brain tumor

Chapter 5   Review Quiz

I. Give meanings for the following combining forms:

1. iatr/o _____
2. nos/o _____
3. onc/o _____
4. orth/o _____
5. esthesi/o _____
6. vascul/o _____

7. rect/o _____
8. pulmon/o _____
9. ur/o _____
10. col/o _____
11. ger/o _____
12. ped/o _____

II. Give combining forms for the following English terms:

1. heart _____
2. voice box _____
3. stomach _____
4. woman _____
5. nerve _____

6. midwife _____
7. mind _____
8. chest _____
9. nose _____

III. Give meanings for the following suffixes:

1. -cele _____
2. -genic _____
3. -scopy _____
4. -stomy _____
5. -therapy _____

6. -tomy _____
7. -megaly _____
8. -algia _____
9. -rrhea _____
10. -osis _____

Chapter 5   Crossword Puzzle Quiz

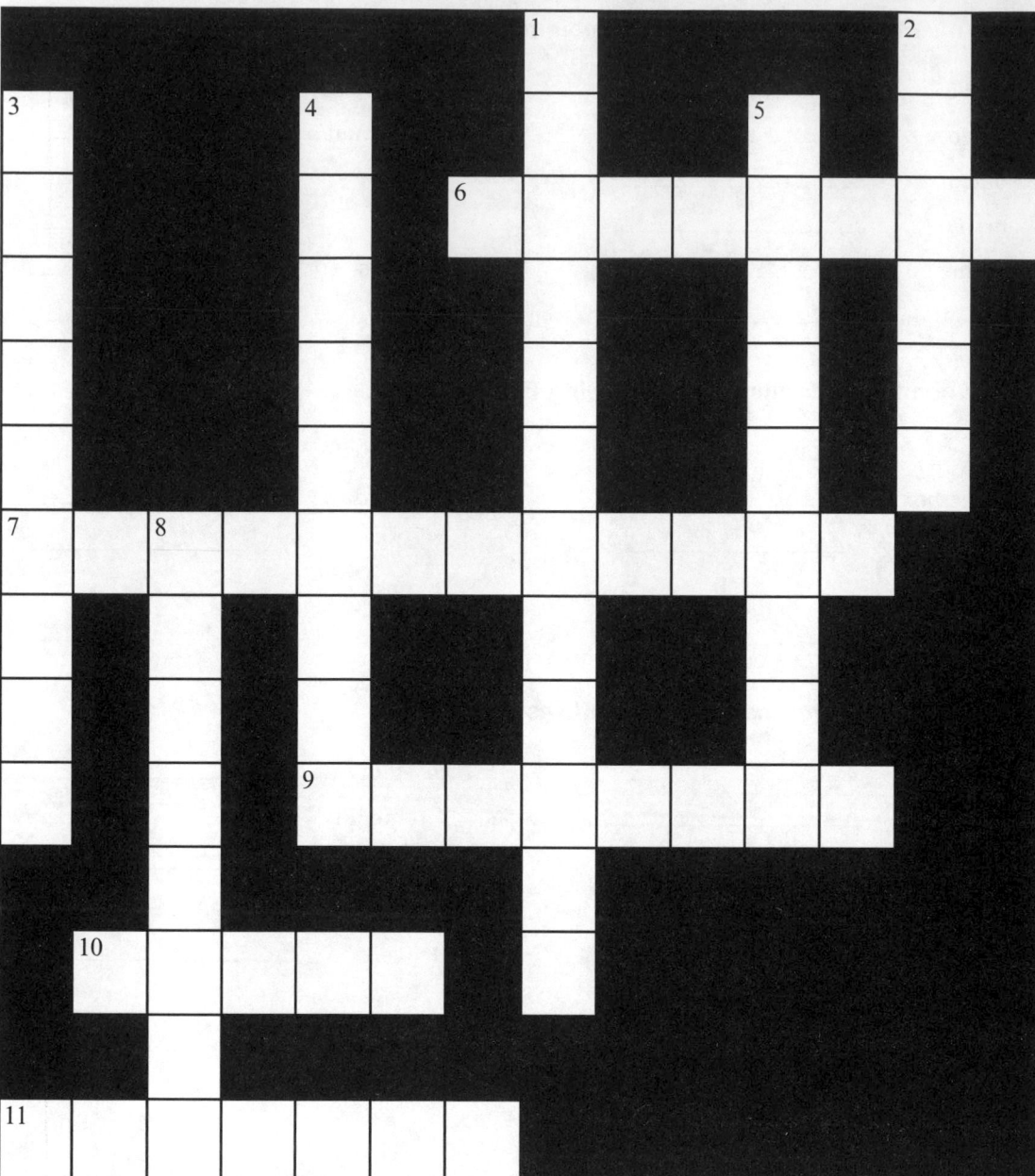

Across

6. combining form meaning *nervous sensation*
7. enlargement of the heart
9. record of sound
10. combining form meaning *treatment*
11. study of the urinary tract

Down

1. resection of the uterus
2. inflammation of the ear
3. hernia of the rectum
4. inflammation of joints
5. pain of the head (headache)
8. combining form meaning *flow* or *fluid* (Hint: think of the area of medicine that treats joint diseases)

Chapter 5   Answers

Multiple Choice Quiz

1. C	11. E
2. E	12. E
3. B	13. E
4. D	14. C
5. E	15. B
6. D	16. D
7. E	17. B
8. C	18. A
9. A	19. B
10. B	20. D

Spelling and Comprehension Quiz

I. Spelling

1. anesthesiology
2. colostomy
3. gastroenterologist
4. gastroscopy
5. geriatrician
6. iatrogenic
7. laryngitis
8. nephrostomy
9. neuralgia
10. obstetrics
11. oncogenic
12. ophthalmologist
13. otitis
14. pathologist
15. pediatrician
16. psychiatrist
17. rectocele
18. rhinorrhea
19. thoracotomy
20. vasculitis

II. Comprehension

2 new opening of the colon to the outside of the body
1 study of administration of agents for loss of sensation
7 inflammation of the voice box
9 pain of nerves
13 inflammation of the ear
6 pertaining to an adverse condition produced by a treatment or physician
20 inflammation of blood vessels
16 physician who treats the mind and mental illness
3 physician who treats disorders of the digestive system
17 hernia of the rectum
11 pertaining to producing a tumor
19 incision of the chest
16 physician who studies disease (reading biopsies and performing autopsies)
4 process of visual examination of the stomach
8 new opening of the kidney to the outside of the body
18 discharge of fluid (mucus) from the nose
10 treatment of pregnant women and delivery of babies
15 physician who treats diseases of children
5 physician who treats diseases of old age
12 physician who treats disorders of the eye

III. Matching

1. E
2. C
3. G
4. J
5. F
6. I
7. A
8. B
9. H
10. D

Review Quiz

I. 1. treatment
2. disease
3. tumor
4. straight
5. sensation
6. blood vessels
7. rectum
8. lung
9. urinary tract
10. colon
11. old age
12. child

II. 1. cardi/o
2. laryng/o
3. gastr/o
4. gynec/o
5. neur/o
6. obstetr/o
7. psych/o
8. thorac/o
9. rhin/o

III. 1. hernia
2. produced by or in
3. process of visual examination
4. opening
5. treatment
6. incision
7. enlargement
8. pain
9. flow; discharge
10. abnormal condition

Crossword Puzzle Quiz

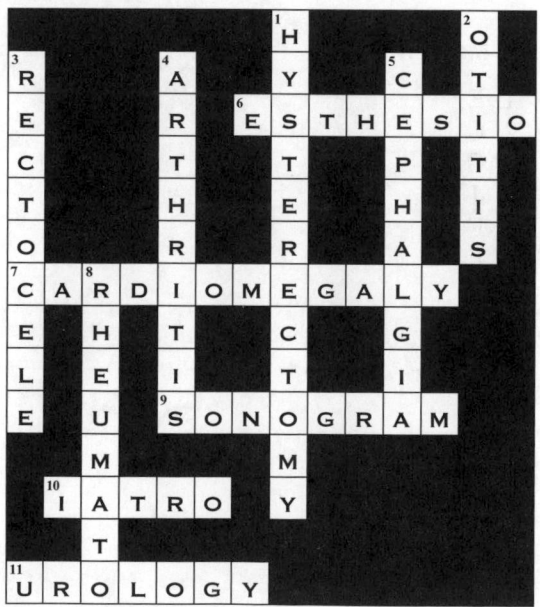

Dictation Sentences

Medical terms that are in **bold** are found in the chapter. Italicized terms may be new to students. Their definitions follow the paragraph.

1. Nosocomial Infections

Nosocomial infections are hospital-acquired infections. They arise at least 72 hours after hospitalization and are most often caused by bacteria, such as *E. coli* or *staphylococci*. Viral causes are the hepatitis viruses or herpes zoster virus. An **infectious disease** specialist often diagnoses and treats nosocomial infections.

   staphylococci: berry-shaped bacteria in clusters

2. Internal Medicine Specialists

An internal medicine specialist, such as a **cardiologist, endocrinologist, hematologist, oncologist, nephrologist, neurologist,** or **rheumatologist,** completes an internal medicine hospital residency after medical school. Following residency, the internist begins a 2- to 3-year fellowship program in a specialty. This includes both **clinical** and **research** training.

3. Surgical Specialists

Surgical specialists include **thoracic surgeons, neurosurgeons, orthopedists, urologists,** and **cardiovascular surgeons.** These doctors complete **surgical** residencies after medical school, and then finish their training with hospital programs in their specialties. The programs focus on **clinical** and **research** training.

4. Eye Care Specialists

An **ophthalmologist** is a medical doctor who specializes in diagnosis and treatment of eye disorders. This physician examines eyes for correction of vision problems, performs eye surgery, and treats eye disorders with medication. An **optometrist** examines eyes and prescribes glasses or contact lenses. An **optician** does not examine eyes, but orders and fits patients with glasses.

Proficiency Examination

This examination is designed to test student proficiency in Chapters 1 to 5. It includes Multiple Choice (50 questions), True/False (25 questions), Short Answer (25 questions) and a Word Parts Challenge (134 questions). It can be used to test students who study the material on their own or as a final examination after teaching Chapter 1 to 5. Answers to the Proficiency Examination are on pp. 92-95.

Proficiency Exam Multiple Choice

1. A prefix meaning "under," "deficient," or "less than normal" is:
   - A. re-
   - B. hyper-
   - C. trans-
   - D. -emia
   - E. hypo-

2. Visual examination of the urinary bladder:
   - A. cystoscopy
   - B. cytology
   - C. cystogram
   - D. nephroscopy
   - E. cystoscope

3. Ren/o and nephr/o both mean:
   - A. heart
   - B. liver
   - C. blood
   - D. kidney
   - E. intestine

4. Prediction about the outcome of treatment:
   - A. prognosis
   - B. psychosis
   - C. diagnosis
   - D. biopsy
   - E. pathology

5. Nerve pain:
   - A. neural
   - B. arthralgia
   - C. cephalgia
   - D. nueralgia
   - E. neuralgia

6. A cerebrovascular accident (CVA) can be caused by:
   - A. gastritis
   - B. osteitis
   - C. adenosis
   - D. dermatitis
   - E. thrombosis

7. Excessive (more than normal) amount of sugar in the blood is:
   - A. hypothyroidism
   - B. hyperthyroidism
   - C. hyperglycemia
   - D. hypoglycemia
   - E. hypodermic

8. Incision of the abdomen:
   - A. laparoscopy
   - B. rhinotomy
   - C. laparotomy
   - D. gastrotomy
   - E. gastroscopy

9. Blood protein found in red blood cells:
   - A. sarcoma
   - B. hemoglobin
   - C. hematoma
   - D. erythrocyte
   - E. hepatoma

10. A malignant (cancerous) tumor of flesh tissue:
    - A. carcinoma
    - B. sarcoma
    - C. neuroma
    - D. hepatoma
    - E. nephroma

11. The voice box is the:
    - A. larynx
    - B. pharynx
    - C. trachea
    - D. esophagus
    - E. bronchial tube

12. The endocrine gland located at the base of the brain is the:
    - A. adrenal gland
    - B. prostate gland
    - C. pituitary gland
    - D. thyroid gland
    - E. pancreas

13. Nervous tissue surrounded by backbones is the:
    - A. vertebrae
    - B. spinal column
    - C. spinal cord
    - D. pelvis
    - E. brain

14. The membrane surrounding the organs in the abdomen is the:
    - A. peritoneum
    - B. esophagus
    - C. pleura
    - D. diaphragm
    - E. mediastinum

15. The space in the chest containing the heart is the:

A. mediastinum
B. pleural cavity
C. cranial cavity
D. abdomen
E. spinal cavity

16. The plane that divides the body into a right and left side is called:

A. frontal
B. transverse
C. cervical
D. sagittal
E. sacral

17. Flexible connective tissue found between bones at joints is:

A. nervous tissue
B. muscle tissue
C. skin
D. epithelial tissue
E. cartilage

18. A series of x-ray images that show the body in cross section is called:

A. MRI (magnetic resonance imaging)
B. chest x-rays
C. gastroscopy
D. laparoscopy
E. CT scan (computerized tomography)

19. The transverse plane:

A. shows a side view of the body
B. divides the body into front and back portions
C. divides the body into upper and lower portions
D. divides the body into right and left parts
E. cannot be viewed with a CT scan

20. Pertaining to the throat:

A. thoracic
B. pharyngeal
C. esophageal
D. tracheal
E. laryngeal

21. -osis means:

A. inflammation
B. tumor
C. pain
D. abnormal condition
E. visual examination

22. A condition in which blood is held back from an organ:

A. ischemia
B. uremia
C. hematuria
D. leukemia
E. menorrhea

23. A benign tumor of muscle is a(an):

A. adenoma
B. adenocarcinoma
C. myoma
D. myosarcoma
E. myocardial infarction

24. Renal failure leads to this blood condition:

A. vasculitis
B. cystitis
C. menorrhagia
D. thrombosis
E. uremia

25. A cancerous tumor of glandular (epithelial) cells is a(an):

A. leukemia
B. hematuria
C. adenoma
D. adenocarcinoma
E. sarcoma

26. A myocardial infarction is a(an):

A. stroke
B. heart attack
C. disease of the brain
D. enlargement of the liver
E. inflammation of a joint

27. Surgical puncture to remove fluid from the sac around the fetus is:

A. arthrocentesis
B. arteriosclerosis
C. hysterectomy
D. laparotomy
E. amniocentesis

28. Removal of pharyngeal lymph tissue:
   A. tonsillectomy
   B. mastectomy
   C. nephrectomy
   D. neurotomy
   E. tracheotomy

29. Separation of waste (urea) from the blood by filtration through a machine:
   A. electroencephalography
   B. arthrocentesis
   C. peritoneal dialysis
   D. abdominocentesis
   E. hemodialysis

30. Combining form for blood vessel:
   A. angi/o
   B. erythr/o
   C. hem/o
   D. leuk/o
   E. arthr/o

31. Before birth:
   A. antigen
   B. antepartum
   C. postpartum
   D. postnatal
   E. neonatal

32. Slow heartbeat:
   A. bradycardia
   B. tachypnea
   C. cardiomegaly
   D. myocardial infarction
   E. tachycardia

33. A protein made by white blood cells and capable of destroying bacteria and viruses:
   A. antibody
   B. antibiotic
   C. antigen
   D. hemoglobin
   E. leukocyte

34. An irregularity that occurs at birth:
   A. intrauterine
   B. neonatal
   C. benign
   D. congenital anomaly
   E. ectopic pregnancy

35. Endocrine glands that are near (above) each kidney:
   A. adrenal
   B. prostate
   C. subcostal
   D. parathyroid
   E. transurethral

36. Poly- has a similar meaning to:
   A. re-
   B. dys-
   C. syn-
   D. hyper-
   E. hypo-

37. A group of symptoms that occur together is a(an):
   A. analysis
   B. syndrome
   C. dialysis
   D. prognosis
   E. remission

38. Process of recording sound waves to make an image of organs in the body:
   A. CT scan
   B. ultrasonography
   C. MRI
   D. endoscopy
   E. dialysis

39. If an organ slides or falls forward, the condition is called:
   A. neoplasm
   B. relapse
   C. remission
   D. prolapse
   E. dysmenorrhea

40. Two prefixes that mean "within":
   A. ante- and pro-
   B. extra- and ec-
   C. hypo- and sub-
   D. syn- and con-
   E. endo- and intra-

41. A specialist who treats glandular disorders is a(an):
   A. gastroenterologist
   B. rheumatologist
   C. endocrinologist
   D. hematologist
   E. otolaryngologist

42. A doctor trained to treat eye disorders is an:
    A. oncologist
    B. optician
    C. optometrist
    D. orthopedist
    E. ophthalmologist

43. A surgeon specializing in disorders of the male reproductive system and urinary tract in males and females:
    A. nephrologist
    B. urologist
    C. gynecologist
    D. neurosurgeon
    E. colorectal surgeon

44. A doctor specializing in treatment of diseases using high-energy radiation:
    A. geriatrician
    B. pathologist
    C. radiologist
    D. radiation oncologist
    E. dermatologist

45. A doctor who specializes in operating on the chest:
    A. thoracic surgeon
    B. colorectal surgeon
    C. otolaryngologist
    D. orthopedist
    E. oncologist

46. Which doctor specializes in treating older patients?
    A. family medicine specialist
    B. geriatrician
    C. rheumatologist
    D. pediatrician
    E. obstetrician

47. A disorder unexpectedly caused by treatment previously prescribed by a doctor is called:
    A. neuralgic
    B. neurogenic
    C. oncogenic
    D. carcinogenic
    E. iatrogenic

48. An opening from the kidney to the outside of the body is a:
    A. nephrostomy
    B. tracheostomy
    C. laparotomy
    D. colostomy
    E. thoracotomy

49. Clinical means:
    A. pertaining to time
    B. pertaining to the lung
    C. pertaining to patient care
    D. pertaining to skin disorders
    E. pertaining to laboratory research

50. Which term is *not* spelled correctly?
    A. laryngeal
    B. pulmonery
    C. vasculitis
    D. neuralgia
    E. gastroenterology

True or False

1.	A doctor who performs autopsies and biopsies is an oncologist.	True	False
2.	A gastrectomy is a gastric resection.	True	False
3.	Record of the electricity in the brain is an electrocephalogram.	True	False
4.	A cancerous tumor of bone marrow is anemia.	True	False
5.	A platelet is an erythrocyte.	True	False
6.	Anterior refers to the back side of the body.	True	False
7.	Epithelial cells line the inner and outer surfaces of the body.	True	False
8.	A backbone is an intervertebral disk.	True	False
9.	The tailbone is the sacrum.	True	False
10.	The tube leading from the urinary bladder to the outside of the body is the urethra.	True	False
11.	An acute condition continues over a long period of time.	True	False
12.	Surgical repair (augmentation or reduction) of breast tissue is mammoplasty.	True	False
13.	Hysterectomy is removal of the uterus, ovaries, and fallopian tubes.	True	False
14.	A myelogram is an x-ray record of the bone marrow after injection of contrast.	True	False
15.	Cystitis is inflammation of a cell.	True	False
16.	The neonatal ICU is for treatment of newborns.	True	False
17.	A subdural hematoma is a malignant tumor.	True	False
18.	Ectopic pregnancies most often occur in the fallopian tubes.	True	False
19.	A spinal cord injury at the lumbar level can lead to hemiplegia.	True	False
20.	When a patient experiences a relapse, all symptoms of the disease disappear.	True	False
21.	Nosocomial infections arise as a result of hospital procedures.	True	False
22.	A rheumatologist is a specialist in allergies and infectious diseases.	True	False
23.	An optometrist can prescribe glasses and contact lenses and medications for eye disorders.	True	False
24.	A pathologist performs autopsies and examines biopsy samples.	True	False
25.	A urologist normally operates to resect a colon and create a colostomy.	True	False

88

Short Answer

1. An increase in malignant white blood cells is a condition called _____.

2. The thyroid gland is an example of a(an) _____ gland.

3. Inflammation of the stomach and small intestine is called _____.

4. Deficiency of hemoglobin in red blood cells is a condition known as
_____.

5. The instrument to visually examine the eye is the _____.

6. Visual examination of the abdomen performed with small incisions and an endoscope
is called _____.

7. Inflammation of the membrane surrounding the lungs is called _____.

8. The muscle separating the thoracic and abdominal cavities is the
_____.

9. An incision of the skull is a(an) _____.

10. The hard backbones in the region of the neck are the _____
_____ (two words).

11. After a sonogram revealed stones in the gallbladder, Mr. Smith was scheduled for a
gallbladder resection or _____.

12. Physicians performed an emergency _____ to make a new opening in
Ms. Jones' windpipe when she choked on a chicken bone.

13. Sarah Settle's oncologist prescribed intensive drug treatment known as
_____ for her breast cancer.

14. Eating foods high in cholesterol and fats can cause collection of fatty plaque in
arteries. This condition is known as _____.

15. Surgical repair to open blocked vessels with a balloon and stent is
_____.

16. During sleep, if a person is momentarily unable to contract respiratory muscles or
maintain air flow through the nose and mouth, it is called sleep _____.

17. A skeletal muscle may undergo _____ as a result of lack of physical
exercise, or neurological or muscular disease.

18. The membrane surrounding a bone is the _____.

19. Biopsy of lymph nodes after Carla's mastectomy revealed three positive axillary
nodes. The pathology report indicated that there was a(an) _____
(spread) of the primary beast cancer.

20. After Carl's leg was amputated to resect an osteosarcoma, he was fitted with an
artificial leg known as a(an) _____.

21. The kidneys lie behind the abdominal cavity in the _____ space.

22. When urinating, Ben noticed blood in his urine, a symptom known as
_____.

23. The physician who gives drugs to keep a patient asleep during surgery is a(an)
_____.

24. Treatment of severe mental disorders is the specialty of a medical doctor called a(an)
_____.

25. A physician (gynecologist) who specializes in delivery of babies is a(an)
_____.

Word Parts Challenge

I. Give meanings for the following combining forms:

1. aden/o _____
2. arthr/o _____
3. cephal/o _____
4. cerebr/o _____
5. cyst/o _____
6. dermat/o _____
7. encephal/o _____
8. gastr/o _____
9. hepat/o _____
10. lapar/o _____
11. nephr/o _____
12. neur/o _____
13. oste/o _____
14. rhin/o _____
15. sarc/o _____
16. bronch/o _____
17. cervic/o _____
18. coccyg/o _____
19. crani/o _____
20. esophag/o _____
21. laryng/o _____
22. mediastin/o _____
23. pelv/o _____
24. peritone/o _____
25. pharyng/o _____
26. pleur/o _____
27. thorac/o _____
28. trache/o _____
29. chondr/o _____
30. vertebr/o _____

31. angi/o _____
32. arteri/o _____
33. axill/o _____
34. cardi/o _____
35. cholecyst/o _____
36. col/o _____
37. hemat/o _____
38. hyster/o _____
39. inguin/o _____
40. mamm/o _____
41. mast/o _____
42. mening/o _____
43. my/o _____
44. oophor/o _____
45. ot/o _____
46. phleb/o _____
47. salping/o _____
48. vascul/o _____
49. cutane/o _____
50. cost/o _____
51. ren/o _____
52. ven/o _____
53. urethr/o _____
54. carp/o _____
55. an/o _____
56. pulmon/o _____
57. pneumon/o _____
58. cyt/o _____
59. ophthalm/o _____
60. enter/o _____

90

II. Give combining forms for the following meaning(s). (Hint: a combining form is the root plus the letter "o"). Use a slash between the root and the combining vowel.

For example: life = <u>bi/o</u>

1. sugar _____
2. side _____
3. spinal cord _____
4. bone marrow _____
5. white _____
6. red _____
7. clot _____
8. time _____
9. x-rays _____
10. cold _____

11. drug _____
12. back, behind _____
13. woman, female _____
14. tumor _____
15. disease _____
16. mind _____
17. knowledge _____
18. cancer _____
19. to hold back _____
20. tonsils _____

III. Give suffixes for the following meanings. Place a hyphen (-) before each suffix.

For example: abnormal condition = <u>-osis</u>

1. blood condition _____
2. instrument to visually examine _____
3. tumor, mass _____
4. incision _____
5. protein _____
6. cell _____
7. inflammation _____
8. excision _____
9. study of _____
10. surgical puncture to remove fluid _____
11. record _____
12. urine condition _____

13. enlargement _____
14. surgical repair _____
15. flow, discharge _____
16. new opening _____
17. hardening _____
18. thirst _____
19. breathing _____
20. excessive discharge of blood _____
21. separation, breakdown _____
22. treatment _____
23. pertaining to producing _____
24. hernia _____

IV. Match the following prefixes with their meanings:

A.

Prefixes		Meaning
1. dys-	_____	through, complete
2. hypo-	_____	too much, above
3. retro-	_____	too little, below
4. brady-	_____	before, in front of
5. tachy-	_____	self
6. dia-	_____	painful
7. aut-	_____	together, with
8. hyper-	_____	behind
9. pro-	_____	slow
10. syn-	_____	fast

B.

Prefixes		Meaning
1. sub-	_____	one
2. trans-	_____	between
3. tri-	_____	across
4. bi-	_____	within
5. uni-	_____	four
6. quadri-	_____	under
7. anti-	_____	three
8. ante-	_____	two
9. inter-	_____	against
10. intra-	_____	before

C.

Prefixes		Meaning
1. pre-	_____	above
2. post-	_____	with
3. peri-	_____	bad
4. con-	_____	before
5. epi-	_____	toward
6. ad-	_____	half
7. hemi-	_____	new
8. neo-	_____	change; beyond
9. mal-	_____	surrounding
10. meta-	_____	after

Proficiency Exam Answers Multiple Choice

1. E	26. B
2. A	27. E
3. D	28. A
4. A	29. E
5. E	30. A
6. E	31. B
7. C	32. A
8. C	33. A
9. B	34. D
10. B	35. A
11. A	36. D
12. C	37. B
13. C	38. B
14. A	39. D
15. A	40. E
16. D	41. C
17. E	42. E
18. E	43. B
19. C	44. D
20. B	45. A
21. D	46. B
22. A	47. E
23. C	48. A
24. E	49. C
25. D	50. B

True or False

1. False	14. False
2. True	15. False
3. False	16. True
4. False	17. False
5. False	18. True
6. False	19. False
7. True	20. False
8. False	21. True
9. False	22. False
10. True	23. False
11. False	24. True
12. True	25. False
13. False	

Short Answer

1. leukemia
2. endocrine
3. gastroenteritis
4. anemia
5. ophthalmoscope
6. laparoscopy
7. pleuritis or pleurisy
8. diaphragm
9. craniotomy
10. cervical vertebrae
11. cholecystectomy
12. tracheostomy
13. chemotherapy
14. arteriosclerosis or atherosclerosis
15. angioplasty
16. apnea
17. atrophy
18. periosteum
19. metastasis
20. prosthesis
21. retroperitoneal
22. hematuria
23. anesthesiologist
24. psychiatrist
25. obstetrician

Word Parts Challenge

I. Meanings

1. gland
2. joint
3. head
4. cerebrum or brain
5. urinary bladder or bladder
6. skin
7. brain
8. stomach
9. liver
10. abdomen
11. kidney
12. nerve
13. bone
14. nose
15. flesh
16. bronchi, bronchus, bronchial tube, or bronchial tubes
17. neck
18. tailbone or coccyx
19. skull or cranium
20. esophagus
21. voice box or larynx
22. mediastinum
23. hip or hipbone
24. peritoneum
25. throat or pharynx
26. pleura
27. chest or thorax
28. windpipe
29. cartilage
30. vertebra or backbone
31. blood vessel
32. artery
33. armpit
34. heart
35. gallbladder
36. colon, large bowel, or large intestine
37. blood
38. uterus or womb
39. groin
40. breast
41. breast
42. meninges
43. muscle
44. ovary
45. ear

46. vein
47. fallopian tube
48. blood vessel
49. skin
50. rib
51. kidney
52. vein
53. urethra

54. wrist bones
55. anus
56. lung or lungs
57. lung or lungs
58. cell
59. eye
60. small intestine or small bowel

II. Combining Forms

1. glyc/o or gluc/o
2. later/o
3. myel/o
4. myel/o
5. leuk/o
6. erythr/o
7. thromb/o
8. chron/o
9. radi/o
10. cry/o

11. chem/o
12. poster/o
13. gynec/o
14. onc/o
15. path/o
16. psych/o
17. gnos/o
18. carcin/o
19. isch/o
20. tonsill/o

III. Suffixes

1. -emia
2. -scope
3. -oma
4. -tomy
5. -globin
6. -cyte
7. -itis
8. -ectomy
9. -logy
10. -centesis
11. -gram
12. -uria

13. -megaly
14. -plasty
15. -rrhea
16. -stomy
17. -sclerosis
18. -dipsia
19. -pnea
20. -rrhagia or -rrhage
21. -lysis
22. -therapy
23. -genic
24. -cele

IV. Prefixes

A.

1. painful
2. too little, below
3. behind
4. slow
5. fast

6. through, complete
7. self
8. too much, above
9. before, in front of
10. together, with

B.

1. under
2. across
3. three
4. two
5. one

6. four
7. against
8. before
9. between
10. within

C.

1. before
2. after
3. surrounding
4. with
5. above

6. toward
7. half
8. new
9. bad
10. change; beyond

Appendix I

Body Systems

Appendix I contains information and activities enabling you to expand your teaching to include basic and simple terminology related to each body system. First, there is an illustration of each system with major organs labeled and combining forms given for each organ. These illustrations as transparency masters can be found at the conclusion of this manual and may be photocopied for classroom use or made into overhead acetates for teaching.

In addition to the illustrations, there is a page of information about each body system. This includes combining forms, their meanings, a medical term using each combining form, and a line for students to write the meaning of the medical term. All answers can be checked in the *Glossary of Medical Terms* at the end of the text. Next, each system contains a short list of major pathological conditions pertinent to that system. Explanations are straightforward and simple, with additional, more difficult terms highlighted in boldface. Again, the meanings of all terms may be referenced in the *Glossary of Medical Terms*. This material, as well as information related to diagnostic and treatment procedures, will help as you teach any or all of the body systems.

In this manual, you will find major abbreviations for each system with Matching Exercises to creatively test understanding of the abbreviations. You may test students on the *exact* meaning of each abbreviation separately. Answers to all Abbreviations Matching Exercises are on p. 120. Beginning on p. 121 you will find practical applications for each body system. These are actual medical records, case reports, or medical writing about a particular disease or procedure. They will help students understand the meanings of terms in context. Answers to this activity can be found on p. 132.

I am eager to know if you teach the body systems in your course and whether or not the practical applications and activities are helpful. Please let me know!

Abbreviations by Body System

I. Cardiovascular System

ACE inhibitors	angiotension-converting enzyme inhibitors (used to treat hypertension, prevent heart attacks, and strokes)
ACS	acute coronary syndromes (unstable angina and acute myocardial infarction)
AF	atrial fibrillation (arrhythmia)
AMI	acute myocardial infarction (heart attack)
ASD	atrial septal defect (abnormal opening in wall between the atria; congenital anomaly)
CABG	coronary artery bypass grafting
CCU	coronary care unit
CTNI	cardiac troponin I (released into bloodstream after myocardial infarction)
CHF	congestive heart failure
DVT	deep venous thrombosis
ECG	electrocardiogram
ECHO	echocardiography
ETT-MIBI	exercise tolerance test combined with a radioactive tracer (Sestamibi) scan
HDL	high-density lipoproteins
HTN	hypertension
LVAD	left ventricular assist device (bridge to transplant)
MVP	mitral valve prolapse
PCI	percutaneous coronary intervention (includes PTCA or angioplasty)
PVC	premature ventricular contraction (arrhythmia)
SSCP	substernal chest pain

Matching Exercises—Cardiovascular System

A. **Match the abbreviation in Column I with its description in Column II.**

Column I

1. AMI _____
2. HDL _____
3. MVP _____
4. ACE inhibitors _____
5. CABG _____
6. AF _____
7. DVT _____
8. ECHO _____
9. LVAD _____
10. ECG _____

Column II

A. Ultrasound record of the heart
B. An arrhythmia; upper chamber beats irregularly
C. A bridge to transport; assist device for heart pump
D. Sagging or prolapse of a left-sided heart valve
E. Clot in a deep vein
F. Electrical record of the heart
G. Drugs to treat hypertension
H. Lipoprotein carrying "good" cholesterol
I. Heart attack
J. Surgery to replace clogged arteries supplying blood to the heart muscle

B.

Column I

1. ACS _____
2. ASD _____
3. CCU _____
4. CTNI _____
5. CHF _____
6. ETT-MIBI _____
7. PCI _____
8. PVC _____
9. SSCP _____
10. HTN _____

Column II

A. Pain under the breastbone
B. High blood pressure
C. Angioplasty is an example
D. Unstable angina and heart attack
E. Treadmill test with radioactive tracer
F. Special unit to care for patients with heart problems
G. Heart is unable to pump required amount of blood
H. Congenital anomaly; hole in wall of the heart
I. Protein released into blood after heart attack
J. An arrhythmia; ventricle beats irregularly

II. Digestive System

BE	barium enema
EGD	esophagogastroduodenoscopy
GB	gallbladder
GI	gastrointestinal
GERD	gastroesophageal reflux disease
IBD	inflammatory bowel disease (ulcerative colitis and Crohn disease)
LFTs	liver function tests (AST, ALT, bilirubin, and alkaline phosphates)
NG tube	nasogastric tube
PUD	peptic ulcer disease
TPN	total parenteral nutrition (IV feeding)

Matching Exercise—Digestive System

Column I		Column II
1. LFTs	_____	A. Stomach and intestines
2. BE	_____	B. Organ below the liver; stores bile
3. PUD	_____	C. Intravenous feeding
4. GERD	_____	D. Crohn disease and ulcerative colitis
5. EGD	_____	E. Placement of a tube from the nose into the stomach
6. GB	_____	F. Open sore or lesion in the stomach or intestine
7. NG tube	_____	G. X-ray examination of the colon
8. IBD	_____	H. Bilirubin, AST, ALT; tests of liver function
9. TPN	_____	I. Visual examination of the esophagus
10. GI	_____	J. Reflux esophagitis

III. Endocrine System

ACTH	adrenocorticotropic hormone
ADH	antidiuretic hormone
DM	diabetes mellitus
FBG	fasting blood glucose
GH	growth hormone
FSH	follicle stimulating hormone
RIA	radioimmunoassay (measures hormone levels in blood)
T_4	thyroxine
TFT	thyroid function test
TSH	thyroid-stimulating hormone

Matching Exercise—Endocrine System

Column I

1. T_4 _____
2. DM   _____
3. RIA   _____
4. GH   _____
5. ACTH   _____
6. TSH   _____
7. FBG   _____
8. TFT   _____
9. ADH   _____
10. FSH   _____

Column II

A. Test to measure sugar in the blood after fasting

B. Pituitary hormone that influences the kidney to hold water in the body

C. Pituitary hormone that stimulates ovaries to produce egg cells

D. Thyroxine

E. Pituitary hormone that stimulates growth of joints and bones

F. Pituitary hormone that stimulates the adrenal cortex

G. Test that measures hormone levels in blood

H. Type 1 and Type 2 and forms of this disease

I. Pituitary hormone that stimulates the thyroid gland

J. Test of thyroid function

IV. Female Reproductive System

AB	abortion; premature termination of pregnancy
CS	cesarean section
CX	cervix
D&C	dilation and curettage
DUB	dysfunctional uterine bleeding
IUD	intrauterine device; contraceptive
GYN	gynecology
Pap smear	test for cervical or vaginal cancer
PID	pelvic inflammatory disease; salpingitis
TAH-BSO	total abdominal hysterectomy with bilateral salpingo-oophorectomy

Matching Exercise—Female Reproductive System

Column I

1. PID   ————
2. CX   ————
3. CS   ————
4. Pap smear   ————
5. AB   ————
6. TAH-BSO   ————
7. DUB   ————
8. D&C   ————
9. GYN   ————
10. IUD   ————

Column II

A. Study of women and women's diseases
B. Removal of the uterus, fallopian tubes, and ovaries
C. Removal of infant from uterus via abdominal incision
D. Widening and scraping of the uterus
E. Salpingitis
F. Premature termination of pregnancy
G. Contraceptive device
H. Lower potion of the uterus
I. Abnormal uterine bleeding
J. Examination of cells from the cervix and vagina

V. Lymphatic System

AIDS	acquired immunodeficiency syndrome
ELISA	enzyme-linked immunosorbent assay (test to detect antibodies in AIDS patients)
G-CSF	granulocyte colony-stimulating factor (promotes white blood cell production)
HAART	hyperactive antiretroviral therapy (for AIDS)
HD	Hodgkin disease; a type of lymphoma
HIV	human immunodeficiency virus
HSV	herpes simplex virus
KS	Kaposi sarcoma
PCP	*Pneumocystis carinii* pneumonia
T-4	lymphocyte that is destroyed by HIV (T-cell lymphocyte)

Matching Exercise—Lymphatic System

Column I

1. HD   _____
2. G-CSF   _____
3. AIDS   _____
4. PCP   _____
5. T-4   _____
6. HIV   _____
7. KS   _____
8. HAART   _____
9. HSV   _____
10. ELISA   _____

Column II

A. Virus that causes AIDS

B. Malignant tumor associated with AIDS

C. Combination of drugs used to treat AIDS

D. Virus (herpes) causing blisters

E. Protein that promotes white blood cell production

F. Type of lymphocyte that is attacked by AIDS virus

G. Syndrome associated with suppression of the immune system

H. Test to detect antibodies to HIV

I. Type of lymphoma

J. Pneumonia associated with AIDS (an opportunistic infection)

VI. Male Reproductive System

BPH	benign prostate hyperplasia (or hypertrophy)
DRE	digital rectal examination
GU	genitourinary
PSA	prostate-specific antigen (test for prostate cancer)
STI	sexually transmitted infection (syphilis or gonorrhea)
TRUS	transrectal ultrasound
TUIP	transurethral incision of the prostate gland
TURP	transurethral resection of the prostate gland

Matching Exercise—Male Reproductive System

Column I		Column II
1. STI	_____	A. Blood test to detect prostate cancer cells
2. DRE	_____	B. Resection of the prostate gland through the urethra
3. TRUS	_____	C. Pertaining to the reproductive organs and urinary tract
4. BPH	_____	D. Non-malignant growth of prostate gland tissue
5. GU	_____	E. Incision of the prostate gland
6. PSA	_____	F. Ultrasound imaging of the prostate gland
7. TURP	_____	G. Examination of the prostate gland through the rectum
8. TUIP	_____	H. Syphilis and gonorrhea

110

VII. Musculoskeletal System

ACL	anterior cruciate ligament (of knee)
C-1 to C-7	cervical vertebrae
Ca	calcium
CTS	carpal tunnel syndrome
EMG	electromyography
IM	intramuscular
L-1 to L-5	lumbar vertebrae
NSAID	nonsteroidal anti-inflammatory drug
RA	rheumatoid arthritis
ROM	range of motion
SLE	systemic lupus erythematosus
T-1 to T-12	thoracic vertebrae

Matching Exercise—Musculoskeletal System

Column I

1. ROM _____
2. IM _____
3. SLE _____
4. EMG _____
5. RA _____
6. CTS _____
7. T-1 to T-12 _____
8. Ca _____
9. NSAID _____
10. ACL _____
11. L-1 to L-5 _____
12. C-1 to C-7 _____

Column II

A. Anti-inflammatory drug
B. Lower back vertebrae
C. Ligament in knee
D. Chronic inflammatory disease involving joints, skin, and other organs
E. Mineral in bones
F. Recording of electricity in muscle
G. Vertebrae in the region of the neck
H. Within a muscle
I. Compression of a nerve in the wrist
J. Area in which a limb can move
K. Vertebrae of the chest
L. Chronic disease of painful joints; especially hands and feet

VIII. Nervous System

AD	Alzheimer disease
ALS	amyotrophic lateral sclerosis
CNS	central nervous system
CSF	cerebral spinal fluid
CVA	cerebrovascular accident (stroke)
EEG	electroencephalogram
LP	lumbar puncture
MS	multiple sclerosis
Sz	seizure
TENS	transcutaneous electrical nerve stimulator (device to relieve nerve pain)

Matching Exercise—Nervous System

Column I

1. CVA _____
2. TENS _____
3. MS _____
4. CNS _____
5. Sz _____
6. AD _____
7. CSF _____
8. LP _____
9. ALS _____
10. EEG _____

Column II

A. Brain and spinal cord
B. Record of electricity in the brain
C. Withdrawal of fluid from a space between the membranes surrounding the vertebrae in the lower back
D. Stroke
E. Gradual deterioration of mental capacity
F. Fluid surrounding the brain and spinal cord
G. Device to relieve nerve pain
H. Degenerative disease of motor nervous in spinal cord
I. Destruction of myelin sheath on neurons in the brain
J. Abnormal electrical activity in the brain

IX. Respiratory System

ABGs	arterial blood gases
COPD	chronic obstructive pulmonary disease (chronic bronchitis and emphysema)
CPAP	continuous positive airway pressure (machine aids breathing)
CPR	cardiopulmonary resuscitation
CXR	chest x-ray
DOE	dyspnea on exertion
NSCLC	non-small cell lung cancer
PE	pulmonary embolism
PFTs	pulmonary function
URI	upper respiratory infection

Matching Exercise—Respiratory System

Column I

1. PFTs   _____
2. CXR   _____
3. URI   _____
4. CPR   _____
5. CPAP   _____
6. NSCLC   _____
7. DOE   _____
8. COPD   _____
9. PE   _____
10. ABGs   _____

Column II

A. Machine aids breathing
B. Difficult breathing on exertion
C. A type of lung cancer
D. Blood test to measure oxygen and carbon dioxide
E. Tests measure breathing function of lungs
F. Blood clot in the lung
G. Posterior/anterior and lateral lung x-rays are taken
H. Airway opened breathing restored and circulation restored
I. Infection in the throat or upper airway
J. Chronic bronchitis and emphysema are examples

X. Skin and Sense Organs

AOM	acute otitis media
AS	left ear (auris sinistra)
Derm.	dermatology
EENT	eyes, ears, nose, and throat
OD	right eye (oculus dexter)
PERRLA	pupils equal round reactive to light and accommodation
PE tube	pressure equalizing tube (in ear)
PPD	purified protein derivative (skin test for tuberculosis)
VA	visual acuity
VF	visual field

Matching Exercise—Skin and Sense Organs

Column I		Column II
1. VF	_____	A. Clarity of vision
2. OD	_____	B. Inflammation of the ear
3. VA	_____	C. Placed in the eardrum to equalize pressure
4. AOM	_____	D. Eyes, ears, nose, and throat
5. PE tube	_____	E. Left ear
6. Derm.	_____	F. Skin test for tuberculosis
7. PPD	_____	G. Evaluation of pupils of the eyes
8. AS	_____	H. Right eye
9. PERRLA	_____	I. Study of the skin
10. EENT	_____	J. The area that the eye is able to see

XI. Urinary System

BUN	blood urea nitrogen (blood test of kidney function)
CRF	chronic renal failure
Cysto	cystoscopy
ESWL	extracorporeal shock wave lithotripsy
HD	hemodialysis
IVP	intravenous pyelogram
K^+	potassium; an electrolyte
Na^+	sodium; an electrolyte
UA	urinalysis
UTI	urinary tract infection

Matching Exercise—Urinary System

Column I		Column II
1. K+	_____	A. Visual examination of the urinary bladder
2. IVP	_____	B. Infection within the urinary tract
3. ESWL	_____	C. Progressive loss of kidney function
4. UTI	_____	D. Sodium
5. HD	_____	E. X-ray of the kidney after injecting contrast in a vein
6. Cysto	_____	F. Analysis of urine
7. CRF	_____	G. Blood test to indicate kidney disease
8. BUN	_____	H. Destruction of stones using shock waves
9. Na+	_____	I. Removal of waste materials from the blood using a machine
10. UA	_____	J. Potassium

Answers to Matching Exercises

Cardiovascular System

A.			B.		
1.	I		1.	D
2.	H		2.	H
3.	D		3.	F
4.	G		4.	I
5.	J		5.	G
6.	B		6.	E
7.	E		7.	C
8.	A		8.	J
9.	C		9.	A
10.	F		10.	B

Digestive System

1.	H		6.	B
2.	G		7.	E
3.	F		8.	D
4.	J		9.	C
5.	I		10.	A

Endocrine System

1.	D		6.	I
2.	H		7.	A
3.	G		8.	J
4.	E		9.	B
5.	F		10.	C

Female Reproductive System

1.	E		6.	B
2.	H		7.	I
3.	C		8.	D
4.	J		9.	A
5.	F		10.	G

Lymphatic System

1.	I		6.	A
2.	E		7.	B
3.	G		8.	C
4.	J		9.	D
5.	F		10.	H

Male Reproductive System

1.	H		5.	C
2.	G		6.	A
3.	F		7.	B
4.	D		8.	E

Musculoskeletal System

1.	J		7.	K
2.	H		8.	E
3.	D		9.	A
4.	F		10.	C
5.	L		11.	B
6.	I		12.	G

Nervous System

1.	D		6.	E
2.	G		7.	F
3.	I		8.	C
4.	A		9.	H
5.	J		10.	B

Respiratory System

1.	E		6.	C
2.	G		7.	B
3.	I		8.	J
4.	H		9.	F
5.	A		10.	D

Skin and Sense Organs

1.	J		6.	I
2.	H		7.	F
3.	A		8.	E
4.	B		9.	G
5.	C		10.	D

Urinary System

1.	J		6.	A
2.	E		7.	C
3.	H		8.	G
4.	B		9.	D
5.	I		10.	F

Practical Applications Exercises by Body System

Cardiovascular System

A 70-year-old man is admitted to the hospital with congestive heart failure. He gives a history of angina pectoris of several years' duration, with recent *exacerbation* of symptoms, such as onset of left-sided chest pain after exercise and, occasionally, *dyspnea*. The pain is usually relieved by ceasing the strenuous activity and placing nitroglycerin tablets *sublingually*. Hypertension may increase during the attack, and arrhythmias may occur.

Questions

1. According to this report, the patient has a history of:
   - A. Inability of the heart to pump its required amount of blood
   - B. High blood pressure and abnormal heart beats
   - C. Difficulty taking medicine under his tongue
   - D. Chest pain

2. Which symptoms may have exacerbated recently?
   - A. Strenuous activity and placing pills under the tongue
   - B. Difficult, painful breathing and exercise-induced chest pain
   - C. Increased widening of arteries
   - D. Difficult digestion and spitting up blood

New Terms

dyspnea: difficult, painful breathing

exacerbation: to increase in severity

nitroglycerin: a drug used to dilate (widen) blood vessels

sublingually: pertaining to under the tongue

Digestive System

History and Plan

cc: Leonard Smith, M.D.

Identifying Data: This 72-year-old female presents with a complaint of a biopsy-proven adenocarcinoma of the sigmoid colon at 20 cm.

History of Present Illness: The patient has been noted to have some bright, red bleeding intermittently for approximately 8 months, initially presumable on a *hemorrhoidal* basis. She recently has had intensification of the rectal bleeding but no weight loss, *anorexia*, or obstructive pain. No significant diarrhea or constipation. Some low back pain, probably unrelated.

Recent colonoscopy by Dr. Scoma revealed a large *sessile* polyp, which was partially excised at the 20-cm level, showing *infiltrating* adenocarcinoma at the base.

The patient is to enter the hospital at this time after home antibiotic and mechanical bowel prep, to undergo sigmoid colectomy and possible low anterior *resection*.

Questions

1. The patient appeared at the doctor's office with a previously diagnosed condition of:
   A. Lack of appetite and low back pain
   B. Sigmoid colectomy
   C. Malignant tumor of the colon
   D. Intensive rectal bleeding

2. What procedure did she have recently that diagnosed her condition?
   A. Visual examination of her large intestine
   B. Removal of her sigmoid colon
   C. Low anterior resection of the large intestine
   D. Hemorrhoidectomy

3. What procedure is she scheduled to have done?
   A. Biopsy of the sigmoid colon
   B. Excision of polyp in her colon
   C. Removal of the sigmoid colon and possible excision of additional colonic tissue
   D. Removal of 20 cm of colon, including the sigmoid colon

New Terms

anorexia: loss of appetite
hemorrhoidal: pertaining to swollen, twisted veins in the rectal region
infiltrating: pathological accumulation in tissues of substances not normal to them
sessile: attached by a broad base
resection: removal, excision

Endocrine System

Information on Insulin Pumps

An insulin pump is often referred to as a continuous *subcutaneous* insulin infusion system (CSII). It is a small, lightweight, electromechanical device, usually worn on a belt, in a pocket, or in a holster hidden under clothing. The pump consists of a reservoir, which most patients fill with a specially *buffered*, fast-acting human insulin called Velosulin BR, or alternatively, insulin lispro.

Infusion sets consist of a 24- to 42-inch plastic *catheter* attached by a connector to the pump's reservoir. A needle or plastic *cannula* at the other end of the tubing inserts into subcutaneous tissue.

Pumps imitate the secretion patterns of the pancreas, but they do an imperfect job. Unlike the pancreas, which secretes insulin directly into the *portal* circulation, the pump delivers insulin into subcutaneous tissue based on a set of programmed instructions, so the body does not respond as quickly to the hormone. The device is also unable to measure changes in blood *glucose* levels over time or automatically vary the volume of insulin delivered in response to these changes. The patient must perform these operations herself.

Questions

1. How do insulin pumps deliver insulin to the body?
   A. Directly into the portal circulation
   B. By intravenous injection
   C. Through a tube connected to a blood vessel
   D. Through a tube inserted into tissue under the skin

2. The insulin pump can
   A. Measure changes in blood sugar levels over time
   B. Automatically vary the amount of insulin delivered
   C. Deliver a chemically regulated human insulin into the body
   D. Cause the body to respond more quickly to hormone

New Terms

buffered: acidity and alkalinity of a solution are regulated; set

cannula: a tube for insertion into a cavity or duct; usually containing a trocar, which is a surgical instrument. Following insertion of the cannula and trocar, the trocar is removed and the cannula remains open as a channel for the flow of fluid.

catheter: a tube for removing or injecting fluids

glucose: sugar

portal: pertaining to veins leading into the liver from the pancreatic region

subcutaneous: pertaining to under the skin (cutane/o)

Female Reproductive System

Case Report

A 20-year-old *G1P0* Hispanic female with prenatal care in Los Angeles presented at 23 weeks (5.7 months) by dates with complaint of painful uterine contractions starting on 2/27/93. Patient presented at 1840 hours on 2/28/93. She reports falling on her buttocks approximately 2-3 days before presentation. UCs began 1 day prior to admission. Negative rupture of membranes; (+) *bloody show*. Good fetal movement. No *PIH* or *UTI* symptoms were reported. Past medical history was unremarkable. Social history and family history were negative. Examination revealed a 23-week size uterus and fetus. Patient was admitted and managed. Patient progressed rapidly in labor and delivered a 575-gram male fetus with a single respiratory gasp. Infant subsequently expired. No *resuscitation* was performed secondary to extreme prematurity. Patient's postpartum course was unremarkable and she was discharged to home following MSW consultation with follow-up at clinic in 6 weeks.

Questions

1. Which abbreviation best describes the patient's reproductive history?
   - A. G1P0
   - B. UTI
   - C. MSW
   - D. PIH

2. On the day before admission, the patient had uterine contractions, probably caused by:
   - A. Rupture of her membranes
   - B. Pregnancy induced hypertension
   - C. Discharge of blood from her urethra
   - D. A fall on the lower part of her back

New Terms

bloody show: vaginal discharge of blood-tinged mucus; often means that the cervix has dilated somewhat and the onset of labor is soon.

G1P0: gravida 1 (first pregnancy); para 0 (no viable offspring produced)

PIH: pregnancy-induced hypertension

postpartum: after birth

resuscitation: administering emergency measures to support newborn adaptation to extrauterine life

UTI: urinary tract infection

Lymphatic System

Disease Information

Hodgkin disease is an abnormal condition of lymph nodes with malignant cells occurring in lymph nodes, spleen, and lymphoid tissues generally. It often begins with a cervical node and may spread throughout the body.

The disease is classified according to stages of development of the malignancy. These stages are helpful in prescribing treatment and establishing a prognosis. Stage I means that there is only involvement of a single lymph node or group of nodes. Stage II is involvement of two or more sites on the same side of the diaphragm. Stage III is disease on both sides of the diaphragm and may include the spleen or localized extranodal disease. Stage IV is widespread involvement, such as in the liver, bone morrow, lung, or skin.

Questions

1. Hodgkin disease primarily affects all of the following except:
   - A. Nervous system
   - B. Lymph nodes
   - C. Spleen
   - D. Bone marrow

2. Stage IV disease means that:
   - A. Tumor is located primarily on one side of the diaphragm
   - B. Tumor is on both sides of the diaphragm, and also in the spleen
   - C. Tumor is in a single lymph node or group of nodes
   - D. Tumor includes tissue outside the lymphatic system and involves hepatopathy, osteopathy, myelopathy, and other organs

New Terms

extralymphatic: pertaining to outside the lymph nodes and lymph vessels and lymphoid tissue

extranodal: pertaining to outside the lymph nodes

stages: classifications reflecting the extent of spread of a malignant tumor

Male Reproductive System

Dear Dr. Smith:

At your request, I evaluated Bill Short in consultation on 5/10/98. As you know, Mr. Short is a 58-year-old white male with newly diagnosed prostate carcinoma who was seen for consideration of possible therapeutic *irradiation*.

During a routine annual physical in February 1998, he was found to have an elevated *PSA* of 5.8. His *DRE* revealed a mildly enlarged prostate without specific nodularity. A repeat PSA a few days later was said to be 6.3. The patient was then seen by Dr. Jones, who confirmed the physical examination and treated the patient with a course of Bactrim for 2 weeks, to rule out prostatitis as an etiology for the elevated PSA. After the antibacterial treatment, the PSA was repeated and reported to me as 7.0. Dr. Jones then referred the patient for a transrectal ultrasound and biopsy, which was performed at Mercy Hospital on 4/22/98. The report describes an enlarged prostate and *seminal vesicle*. No focal nodules were seen. The pathology report from Mercy Hospital describes adenocarcinoma, moderately *differentiated*, *Gleason 3 + 3 = 6*.

Questions

1. What blood test led the doctors to suspect that Mr. Short had prostate carcinoma?
    A. DRE
    B. PSA
    C. Gleason score
    D. Transrectal ultrasound

2. What treatment ruled out prostatitis as a possible diagnosis?
    A. Biopsy of the prostate gland
    B. Irradiation of the prostate gland
    C. Two-week course of an antibacterial drug
    D. Seminal vesicle biopsy

New Terms

differentiated: the degree of specialization or maturity of cells composing the tumor; moderately differentiated cells are mid-way between well-differentiated (closest to normal cells) and undifferentiated (most unspecialized and looking like cancer cells).

DRE: digital rectal examination.

Gleason 3 + 3 = 6: this is a grading system for prostate cancer. Grading means assessing the degree of differentiation or specialization of the tumor cells. Cells that are graded as 1 are normal, and those that are graded as 5 are very abnormal (malignant). The first number in the grade is for the most prevalent type of cells, and the second number assesses the next most prevalent type of cell in the tumor mass.

irradiation: use of high-energy radiation to destroy tumor cells.

PSA: prostatic specific antigen; a substance found in the bloodstream; produced both by malignant tumor cells and cells that are inflamed.

seminal vesicle: one of two glands located near the prostate gland; produces semen that is excreted during ejaculation.

Musculoskeletal System

MRI Examination—Consultation Report

Reason for exam: Rupture tendon R. foot

MRI of the Right Ankle

Indication: Ruptured tibialis, posterior tendon

Findings: The examination is correlated with outside plain radiographs performed

1-19-97. The plain radiographs demonstrated flattening of the *plantar arch* and soft tissue swelling over the medial *malleolus*. The MRI examination demonstrates normal signal intensity from the bone marrow spaces. There is a moderate-sized joint *effusion* present. There is increased signal within the substance of the tibialis posterior tendon insertion, and soft tissue *induration* is seen within the surrounding tissues extending into the subcutaneous tissue.

Impression:

(1) There is thickening and increased signal within the tibialis posterior tendon near its insertion, suggestive of a partial intrasubstance tear. There is soft tissue induration in this region.

(2) There is a moderate-size effusion within the ankle joint.

Questions

1. The patient has had an injury to:
    A. Right ankle; outside area
    B. Right ankle; inner region
    C. Left ankle inner process near the fibula
    D. Portion of the knee associated with the tibial bone

2. The MRI indicates that the patient has a:
    A. Ligament tear around the ankle
    B. Fluid collection near the knee
    C. Tumor located near the ankle
    D. Fluid collection over the medial part of the ankle and tear of the connective tissue connecting muscle to bone

New Terms

effusion: escape of fluid into tissue or a part of the body

induration: hardening of tissue; usually due to collection of fluid

malleolus: a rounded process on either side of the ankle joint

plantar arch: curved portion (arch) of the sole (plantar) or bottom of the foot

Nervous System

Medical Report

Nosocomial meningitis is extremely rare in patients who have not undergone neurosurgery. Lumbar puncture is a procedure often used to diagnose meningitis. Because the *morbidity* and cost associated with lumbar puncture are not insignificant, the procedure may often safely be deferred while other possible diagnoses with similar symptoms are examined.

Hospital patients with symptoms such as fever and *delirium* frequently undergo lumbar puncture to decide if meningitis is the correct diagnosis. A recent study showed that none of the lumbar punctures performed on nonsurgical patients to rule out *nosocomial* meningitis yielded an abnormal *CSF*, despite the presence of delirium, headache, and meningeal signs in some of those patients.

Questions

1. According to this report, lumbar puncture is:
    A. Good treatment for meningitis
    B. Always appropriate for diagnosis of hospital-caused meningitis
    C. A type of meningitis that occurs in a hospital
    D. Not always necessary to diagnose hospital-caused meningitis

2. Fever and delirium:
    A. Are often signs of meningitis
    B. Occur after lumbar punctures are performed in a hospital
    C. Are used to rule out nosocomial meningitis
    D. Often indicate that the patient has an abnormal CSF

New Terms

CSF: cerebrospinal fluid (found in ventricles, or chambers, in the brain and between the membranes surrounding the brain and spinal cord)

delirium: acute, fleeting loss of consciousness with change in awareness of surroundings and disorganized thinking

morbidity: condition of being diseased

nosocomial: pertaining to originating in a hospital

Respiratory System

Bronchoscopy Report

Bronchoscopy: left thoracotomy with wedge pulmonary resection of the left lower lobe; mediastinal lymph node biopsy.

Operative Procedure: Once the endotracheal tube was in place, the flexible bronchoscope was used to make a complete endobronchial examination with the findings indicated below. A left posterolateral thoracotomy incision was made and the seventh rib was excised subperiosteally. The pleural space was explored with the findings indicated below. A lymph node was excised and submitted for frozen section. The lesion in the lung was excised using a 30-mm stapling device.

Findings: Bronchoscopy through the endotracheal tube showed a normal distal trachea and *carina,* and the left and right tracheobronchial systems were entirely normal. All the segmental bronchi were widely *patent* inside the chest. One small *adhesion* was present at the *apex* of the pleural space. The lung *parenchyma* immediately beneath this area was mildly scarred. A nodular lesion was found in the subpleural area and the lateral *basilar* segment of the left lower lung. An enlarged lymph node was present and this lesion on frozen section was reported as showing nonspecific inflammation.

Questions

1. The procedure included all of the following except:
    - A. Visual examination of the windpipe and bronchi
    - B. Incision of a bronchus with removal of a rib
    - C. Side and back incision of the chest
    - D. Resection of a lymph node

2. A finding as a result of the procedure was:
    - A. Tumor blocking the right distal bronchi
    - B. Narrowing of some of the bronchi
    - C. Nodular lesion under the pleura at the base of the left lower lobe of the lung
    - D. Lymph node biopsy showed malignancy and inflamed tissue

New Terms

adhesion: union of two surfaces that are normally separate; adhesions are often scar tissue resulting from surgery

apex: pointed end of a structure; the apex of the lung is its uppermost part

basilar: pertaining to the base (lower arm)

carina: a ridge at the lower end of the trachea separating the openings of the two bronchi

parenchyma: the essential parts of an organ that are concerned with its main function

patent: open

Skin and Sense Organs

Case Report

The patient, a 46-year-old female, initially had malignant melanoma diagnosed in April 1986 when she underwent excision of three lesions from her left arm with wide local excision and left *axillary* node dissection. She was first noted to have metastatic disease manifested by a mass in the lower lobe of the right lung on chest x-ray in April 1989. The lesion was resected and she was treated with an experimental immunotherapy *protocol* consisting of melanoma antigen. In November of 1990, the patient developed metastatic disease in her brain and after surgery to remove the mass, the area was *irradiated*.

In early 1991, she developed metastatic disease in her right fibula, right lower lobe of lung, and liver. She was treated with combination chemotherapy consisting of bleomycin, Velban, and cisplatin without positive response. A one-month course of interferon was given, but discontinued because of low *granulocyte* count. *Tamoxifen* therapy was initiated in January of 1992 after metastatic melanoma was found in the membranes of the spinal cord and surgically resected.

Shortly thereafter, she had another brain lesion resected, followed by radiotherapy. She resumed tamoxifen treatment with consequent gradual resolution of several metastatic lesions.

The patient remained essentially stable from 1993 to May 1998 when she developed persistent fatigue. Workup revealed extensive metastatic melanoma in her spleen with subsequent splenic rupture, which required surgical excision of the spleen. Intraperitoneal and liver metastases were noted at that time.

Treatment with biological and chemotherapy failed to affect the relentless spread of the disease, and the patient expired of hepatic failure in September of 1998.

Questions

1. The patient's cancer spread to all the following areas except:
    A. Brain and meninges
    B. Kidney
    C. Spleen and liver
    D. Lung

2. The patient's combination chemotherapy trial consisted of:
    A. Use of several drugs together
    B. Use of radiation to destroy the tumor tissue
    C. Surgical resection of the lesions
    D. Tamoxifen treatment

New Terms

axillary: pertaining to the arm pit (underarm area)

protocol: a plan for treatment

granulocyte: a type of white blood cell

irradiated: use of high-energy radiation to destroy tissue

tamoxifen: drug that has an antiestrogen effect and combats tumor growth in breast and other cancers

Urinary System

Case Study

The patient, a 50-year-old woman, presented herself at the clinic complaining of dysuria. This symptom was followed by sudden onset of hematuria and clots. There had been no history of *urolithiasis*, *pyuria*, or previous hematuria. *Nocturia* was present about 5 years ago. *Panendoscopy* revealed a carcinoma located about 2 cm from the left ureteral *orifice*. A partial cystectomy was carried out and the lesion cleared. A metastatic workup was negative. Bilateral pelvic lymphadenectomy revealed no positive nodes.

Questions

1. The patient's reason for appearing at the clinic was:
    A. Scanty urination
    B. Inability to urinate
    C. Pus in her urine
    D. Painful urination

2. What acute symptom followed?
    A. Vomiting blood
    B. Blood in urine
    C. High levels of urea in the blood
    D. Blood in feces

3. The patient's diagnosis was:
    A. Malignant tumor of the urinary bladder
    B. Tumor in the proximal ureter
    C. Benign tumor of the urinary bladder
    D. Nighttime urination with urinary bladder stones

4. What procedure indicated that the tumor had not spread?
    A. Resection of part of the urinary bladder
    B. Visual examination of the urinary bladder with a wide-angle view
    C. Removal of lymph nodes on both sides of the hip region
    D. Removal of kidney stones

New Terms

nocturia: excessive urination at night

orifice: opening

panendoscopy: visual examination of the interior of an organ with a wide-angle view

pyuria: pus in urine

urolithiasis: abnormal condition of stones in the urinary tract

Answers to Practical Applications

Cardiovascular System

1. D
2. B

Digestive System

1. C
2. A
3. C

Endocrine System

1. D
2. C

Female Reproductive System

1. A
2. D

Lymphatic System

1. A
2. D

Male Reproductive System

1. B
2. C

Musculoskeletal System

1. B
2. D

Nervous System

1. D
2. A

Respiratory System

1. B
2. C

Skin and Sense Organs

1. B
2. A

Urinary System

1. D
2. B
3. A
4. C

V. Classroom-Tested Activities

Here are two types of classroom-tested activities that you may want to try with your students. The first, a spelling bee, is a small-group activity. It was devised by Carole M. Michael from the University of Charleston, Radiography Program, Charleston, West Virginia. I am grateful to Carole for sharing it with us.

The second activity is one that I have used with my own students. At the end of my course, as an extra-credit project, I often ask students to compose their own medical report or vignette, using medical terms. They may relate a medical experience or create one using terms they have learned. I suggest that you try this with your own classes. I am including some stories that my students have written. You may want to show them to your students as examples and as inspiration for their own attempts. Alternatively, you can give your students a list of terms that they should use and incorporate into a story. For example, directions to students might be: Write a short medical vignette using the following terms correctly in sentences (coronary arteries, ischemia, arteriosclerosis, thrombosis, angiogram, angioplasty, myocardial infarction).

I am sure there are many more interesting activities that you are using in your own classrooms. I hope that you will write to me with your ideas, so that others may benefit in the next edition of this text and Instructor's Manual.

Spelling Bee

Created by Carole Michael

Directions

Have the class divide up into groups of three. Each group will consist of the following:

- 1 person designated as "caller"
- 1 person designated as "speller"
- 1 person designated as "scorekeeper"

Each group will be given three blank score cards and three different lists of medical terms already covered in class. The caller will pronounce the terms on one of the lists. The speller will spell the terms AND give their meanings. The scorekeeper will score the speller's responses as follows:

- +2 points for each correct spelling AND meaning
- –2 points for each incorrect spelling AND meaning
- +1 point for each correct spelling but incorrect meaning
- +1 point for each correct meaning but incorrect spelling

Students will switch roles and lists every 10 minutes. Instructor is timekeeper.

NOTE: The speller may need to appeal to the instructor if he or she thinks the caller is mispronouncing a term.

Materials Needed

- Timer
- Tally sheets (you can photocopy next page)
- Word lists (you can photocopy completed exercises like the Pronunciation of Terms lists from *Medical Terminology: A Short Course* and use these or make your own from the *Glossary of Medical Terms.*)

NOTE TO THE INSTRUCTOR: I use a timer with a bell or buzzer instead of my watch to keep time so that I can mingle around the classroom and act as a facilitator when the need arises. Also, I can monitor individual student's strengths and weaknesses and modify future activities based on my observations. You can modify the activity for different group sizes. For example, a group of four people would allow one person to time responses and keep them within one or two minutes for each term.

Spelling Bee Score Card

Speller: _____

Caller: _____

Scorekeeper: _____

Date: _____

	Correct Spelling and Meaning (+2)	Incorrect Spelling and Meaning (−2)	Correct Spelling Only (+1)	Correct Meaning Only (+1)
1st term				
2nd term				
3rd term				
4th term				
5th term				
6th term				
7th term				
8th term				
9th term				
10th term				
11th term				
12th term				
13th term				
14th term				
15th term				
16th term				
17th term				
18th term				
19th term				
20th term				
Totals				
GRAND TOTAL (add all four columns)				

Student-Created Medical Stories

1. Gastrointestinal Case

A 32-year-old man was experiencing chronic severe pain extending from the right and left upper quadrants into the epigastric region and there was no evidence of internal bleeding. A history was taken.

He had been taking Zantac, Tagamet, and other ulcer-treating medications for the past three years. He was currently on Tagamet—two tablets 150 mg each, b.i.d. This level of medication was no longer effective. An endoscopy was scheduled and an emergency colonoscopy was performed. The fiberoptic colonoscope was introduced and was continued for almost 36 inches. No neoplasms were detected. The colonoscope was withdrawn.

A previous endoscopy, two years earlier, had shown no abnormal growths. A confirmatory barium swallow was conducted. No ulcers were detected. The original diagnosis of hiatal hernia was reconfirmed. He was also scheduled for a barium enema.

The patient prepared for the barium enema with a forty-eight hour solid food fast, with no liquids after the first twenty-four hours. He came into the lab in good spirits, despite the length of time without nourishment. He did not tolerate the procedure well, but the technicians were able to complete it in full.

The patient was advised to take the following steps:

- Drink no caffeine
- Increase the height of his head while sleeping by elevating that end of the mattress
- Eat nothing after 9:00 PM at night

2. My Cesarean Section

I was brought to labor and delivery. Immediately, the nurse placed the fetal monitor across my abdomen to record my infant's heart rate. Due to the fact that I previously had a cesarean section, the nurses began to prep me for surgery to have a repeat c-section. I was given an epidural to numb the abdomen from the waist down. The orderly then moved me to the surgery room.

The doctor made a transverse incision in the lower part of my abdomen. Then she carefully removed the fetus and placed it on my abdomen. Next she cut the umbilical cord. The infant was then given to the pediatric team for the Apgar score evaluation—to check heart rate, respiration, color, muscle tone, and reflex. In the meantime, the doctor removed the placenta, which is also known as the "afterbirth." She then began sewing where the incision was made. I was moved to the recovery room for two hours. The nurses then gave me injections of Demerol for the pain. The orderly moved me to my room for further hospital care.

3. An Infectious Disease Story

Four years ago, I developed a bacterial infection in my pharynx. My symptoms included dysphagia, lymphadenitis, and dehydration. When the doctor examined me, he palpated my abdomen and took a sample of blood to test for mononucleosis. My condition was idiopathic. The doctor prescribed an antibiotic and advised me to start getting some fluids in my body or I would have to be hospitalized and fed intravenously. Fortunately, the antibiotic that he prescribed fought off the infection and within two days I was feeling much better.

4. Donny's Hernia

At my son Donny's third month checkup visit, his pediatrician noticed a small hernia in the right side of his groin. He suspected that it might be an inguinal hernia. He referred me to a general surgeon for a second opinion. After examining Donny, the general surgeon diagnosed Donny as having an inguinal hernia. He said that surgery would be needed to perform a herniorrhaphy.

His prognosis was that Donny would recover quickly and would get through the surgery just fine. The surgeon said that the surgery didn't have to be done right away even though the hernia was very painful and would enlarge rapidly. He also told us that the hernia would begin making a gurgling noise due to part of his intestine protruding into the groin region. The surgery was done very soon thereafter. But, again, at my son's 13-month checkup visit, his pediatrician noticed a hernia on the other side of his groin. He referred me again to the same general surgeon, who performed the herniorrhaphy once again. My son is now 14 years old and has never since had any related problems.

5. A Gynecologic Visit

Last month I visited a new gynecologist (female) after having a male gynecologist for many years. Since new patients are required on initial visits to submit their medical history, I have listed below, in part, my medical history:

- Gravida 3, Para 3
- Cesarean section
- Tubal ligation
- Cysts removed from an ovary
- Benign cyst removed from left breast
- Hysterectomy

First, the gynecologist performed a Papanicolaou test (Pap smear). This procedure was performed by opening my vagina with a speculum and then collecting cells scraped from my cervix and vagina (to examine this for abnormalities). Next, the gynecologist examined my breasts and referred me to the radiology department for a mammogram.

The radiologist explained the mammography procedure and said that I would feel some pressure. She added that some women were very sensitive and felt a lot of pain. She then took various x-rays of my breasts and axilla. Fortunately, I did not have pain during this procedure.

I received negative results on the mammogram, but the results of the Pap smear from the pathologist are not available at this time. I am confident that the examination will also be negative.

VI. Transparency Masters

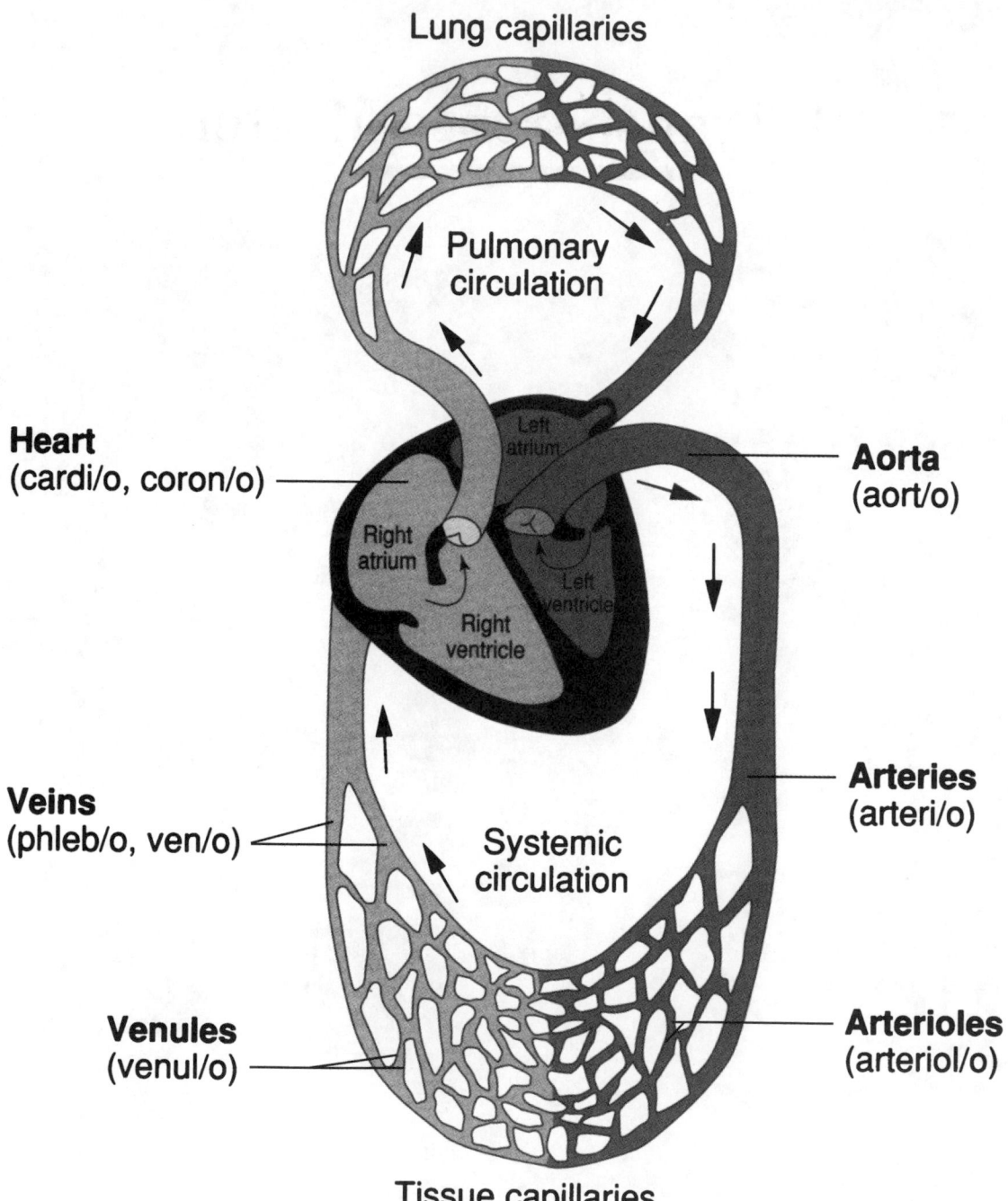

Lung capillaries

Pulmonary circulation

Heart
(cardi/o, coron/o)

Left atrium

Right atrium

Left ventricle

Right ventricle

Aorta
(aort/o)

Arteries
(arteri/o)

Veins
(phleb/o, ven/o)

Systemic circulation

Venules
(venul/o)

Arterioles
(arteriol/o)

Tissue capillaries

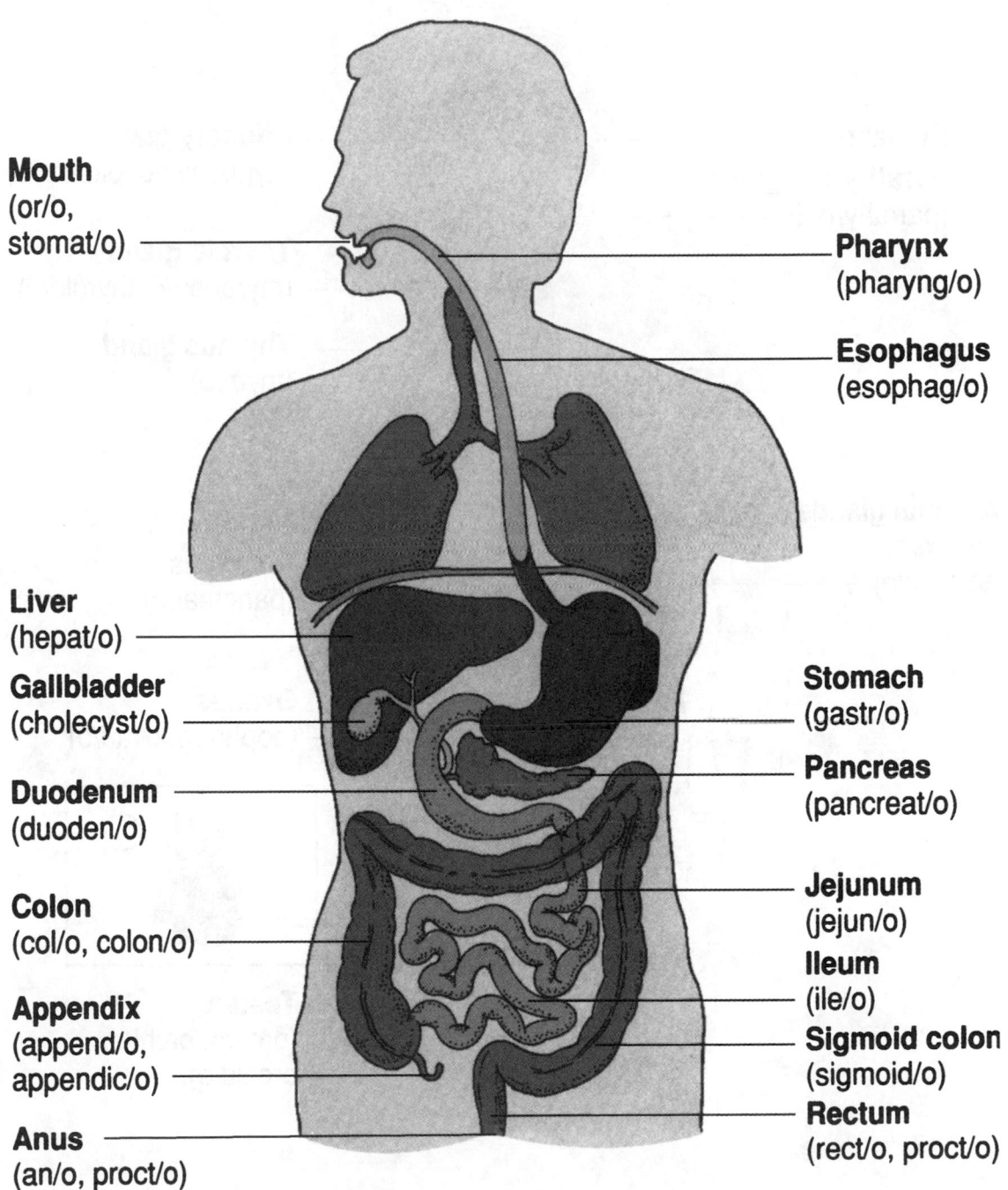

Mouth
(or/o,
stomat/o)

Pharynx
(pharyng/o)

Esophagus
(esophag/o)

Liver
(hepat/o)

Gallbladder
(cholecyst/o)

Duodenum
(duoden/o)

Colon
(col/o, colon/o)

Appendix
(append/o,
appendic/o)

Anus
(an/o, proct/o)

Stomach
(gastr/o)

Pancreas
(pancreat/o)

Jejunum
(jejun/o)

Ileum
(ile/o)

Sigmoid colon
(sigmoid/o)

Rectum
(rect/o, proct/o)

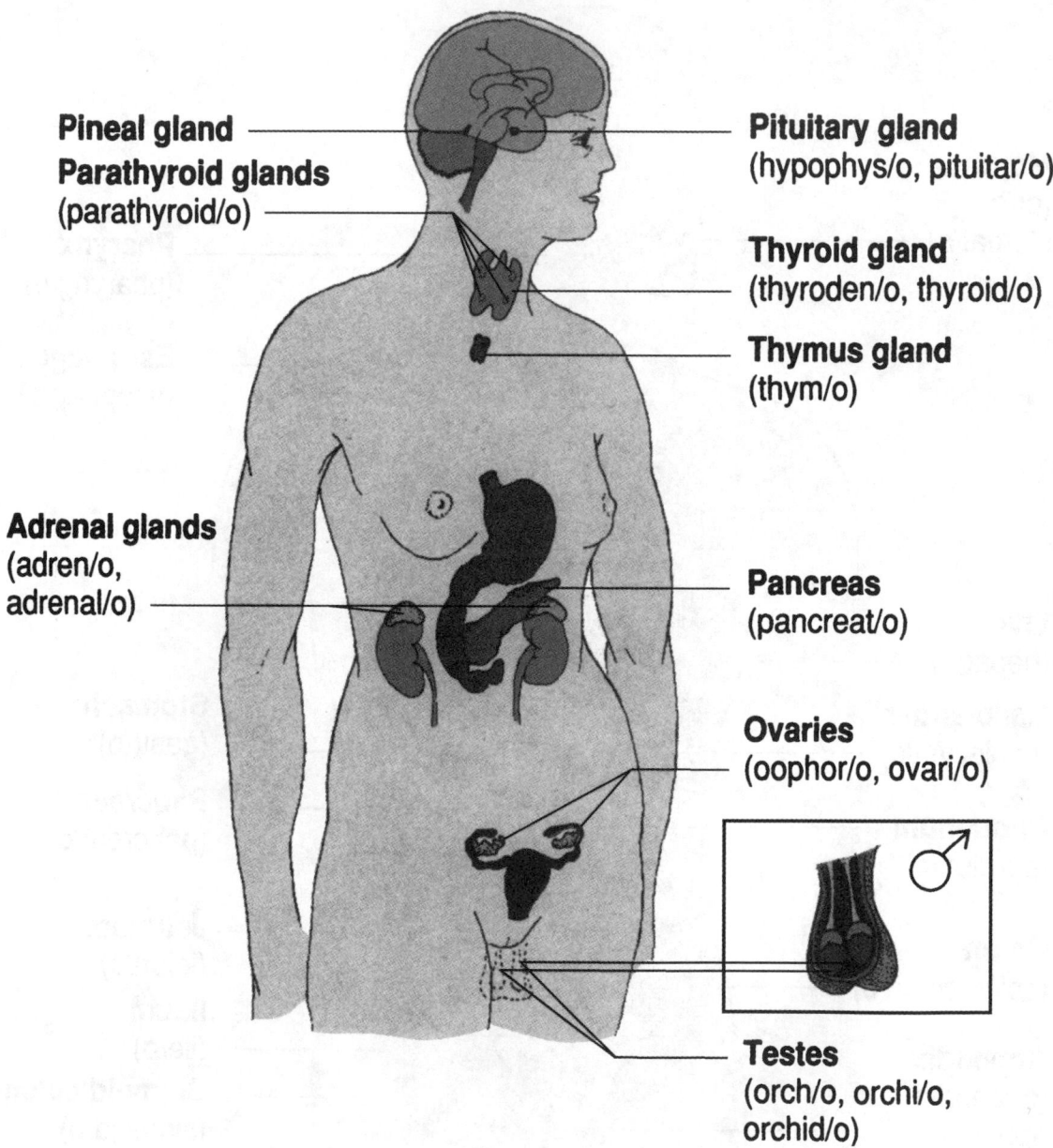

Pineal gland

Parathyroid glands
(parathyroid/o)

Pituitary gland
(hypophys/o, pituitar/o)

Thyroid gland
(thyroden/o, thyroid/o)

Thymus gland
(thym/o)

Adrenal glands
(adren/o,
adrenal/o)

Pancreas
(pancreat/o)

Ovaries
(oophor/o, ovari/o)

Testes
(orch/o, orchi/o,
orchid/o)

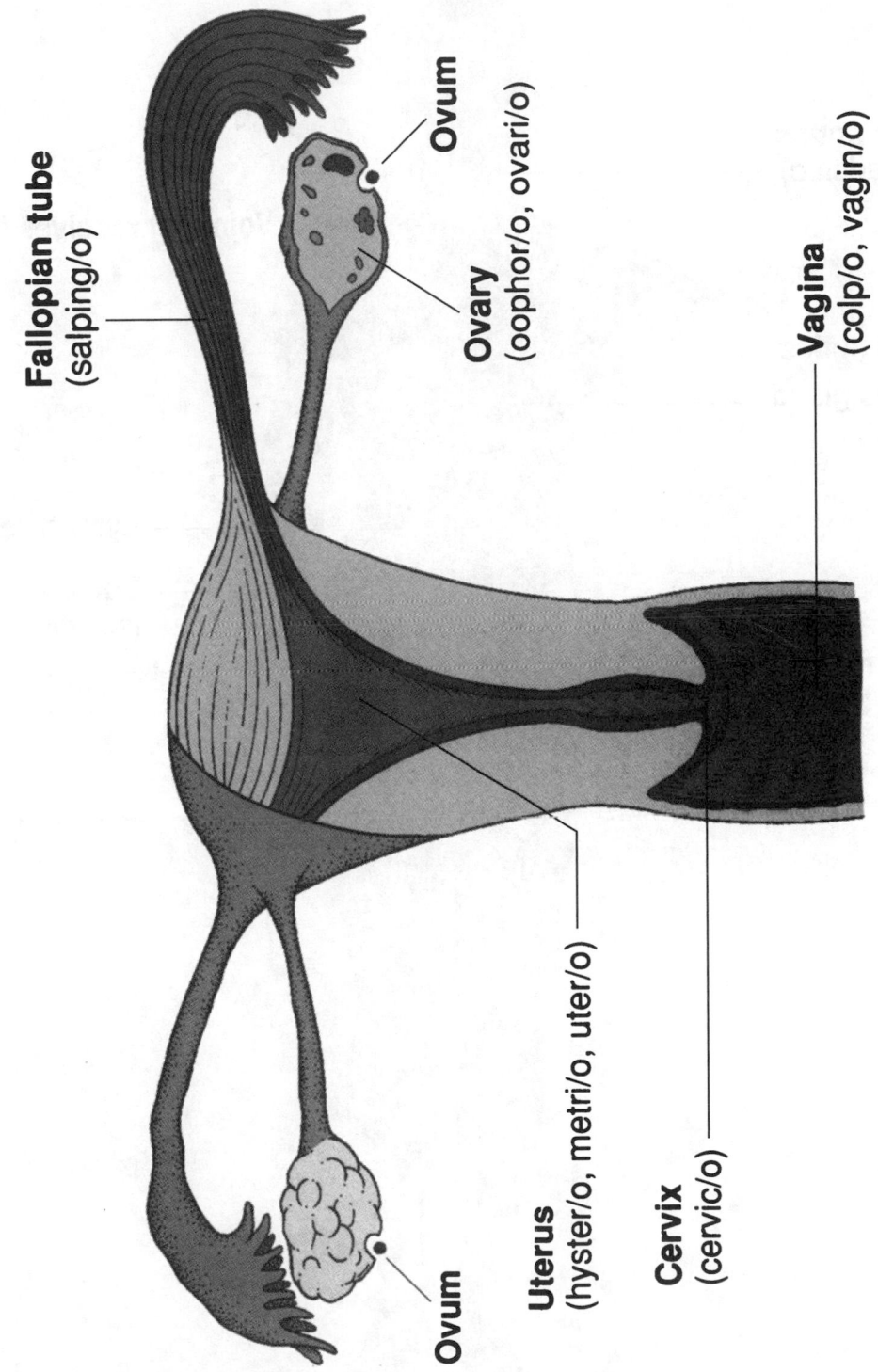

Fallopian tube
(salping/o)

Ovum

Ovary
(oophor/o, ovari/o)

Vagina
(colp/o, vagin/o)

Uterus
(hyster/o, metri/o, uter/o)

Cervix
(cervic/o)

Ovum

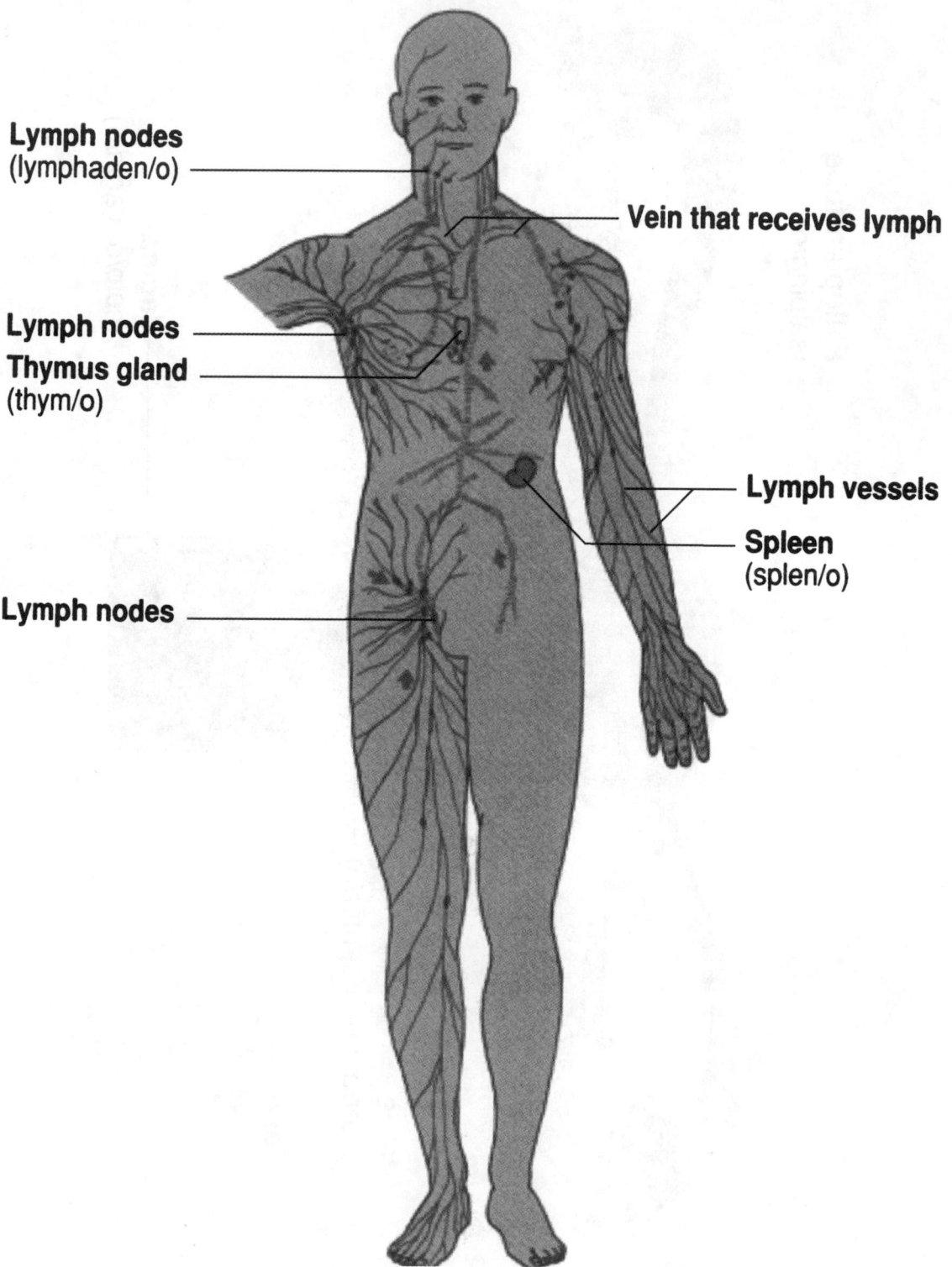

Lymph nodes
(lymphaden/o)

Vein that receives lymph

Lymph nodes

Thymus gland
(thym/o)

Lymph vessels

Spleen
(splen/o)

Lymph nodes

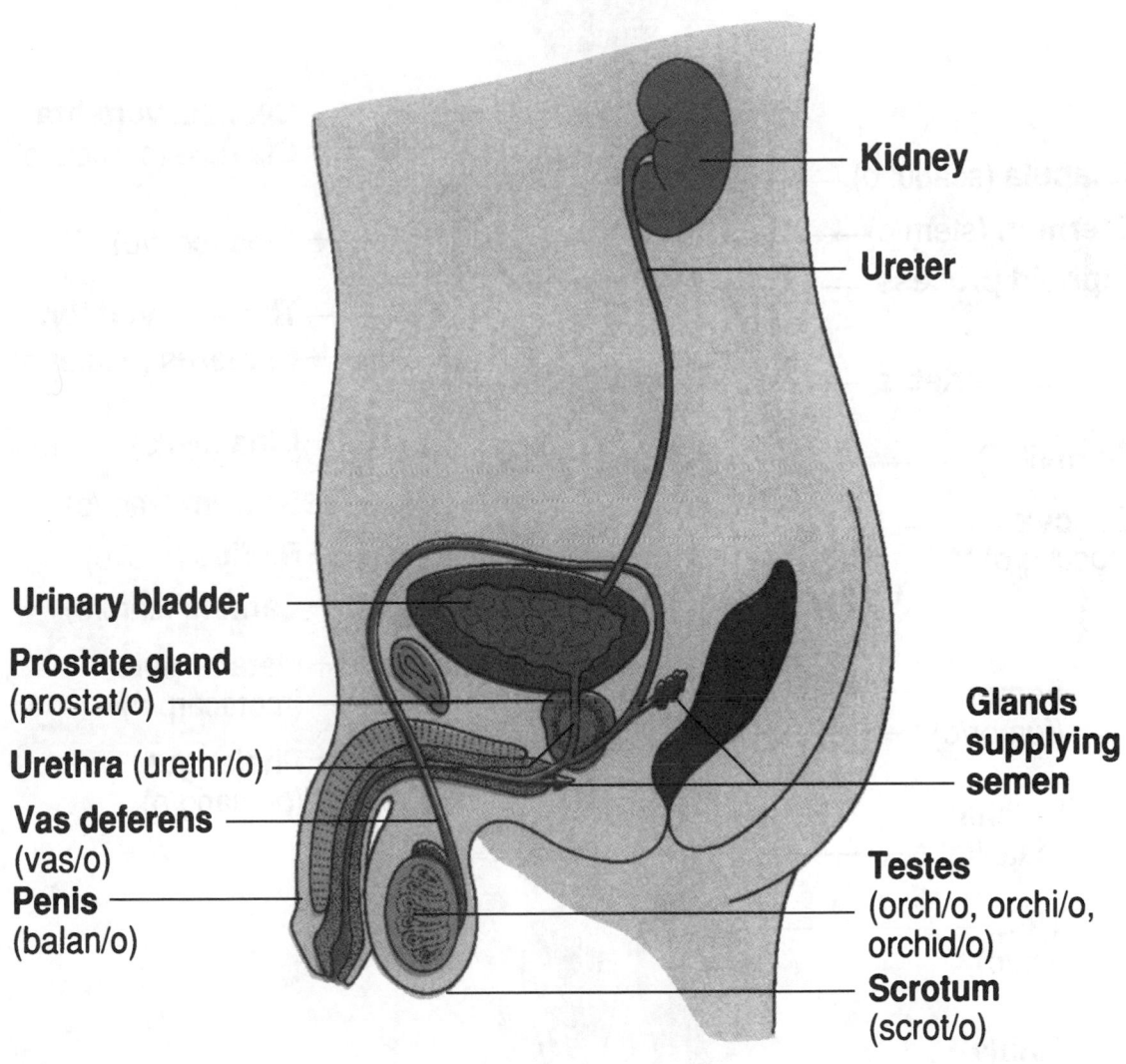

Kidney

Ureter

Urinary bladder

Prostate gland
(prostat/o)

Urethra (urethr/o)

Vas deferens
(vas/o)

Penis
(balan/o)

Glands supplying semen

Testes
(orch/o, orchi/o, orchid/o)

Scrotum
(scrot/o)

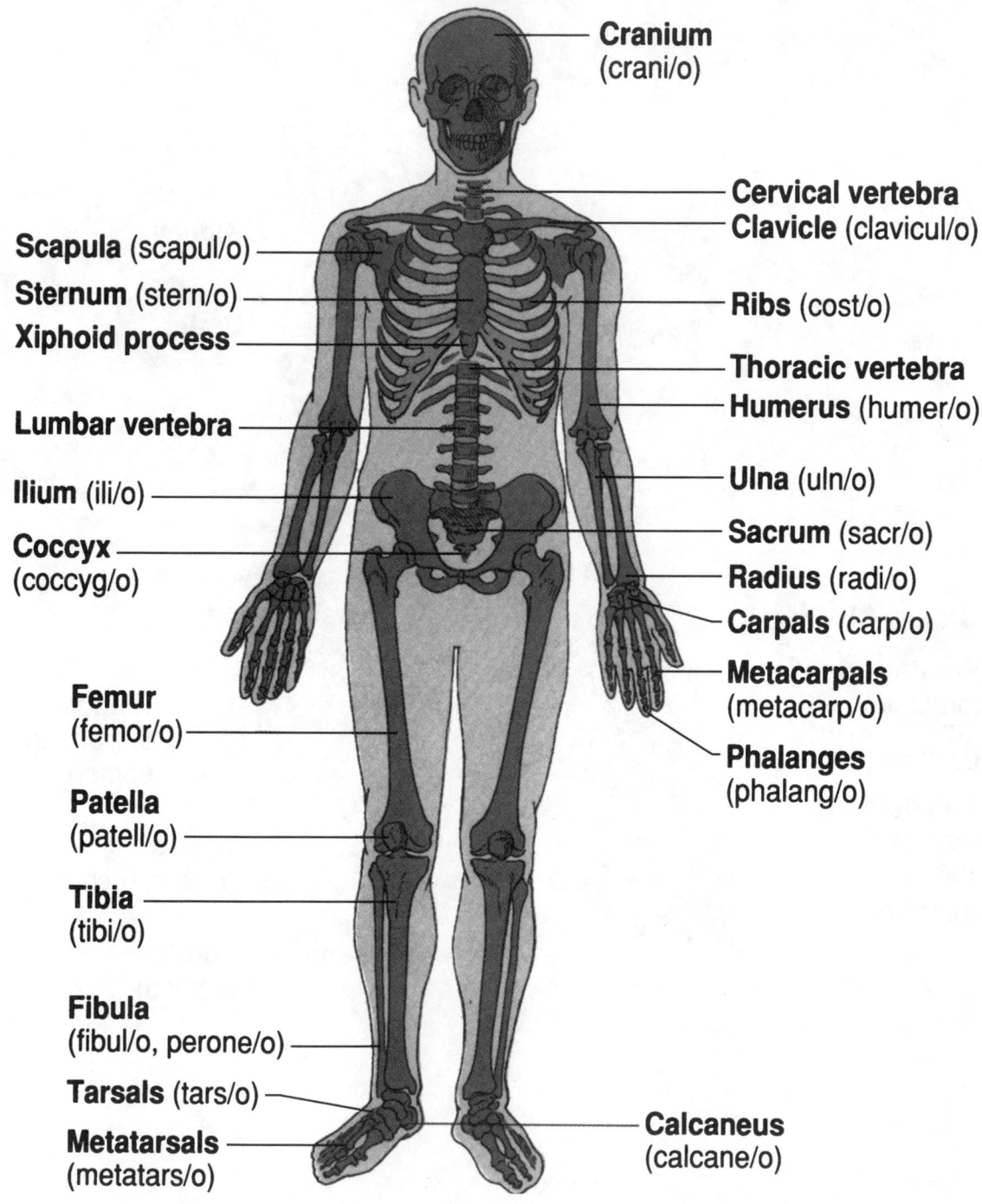

Cranium (crani/o)

Cervical vertebra

Clavicle (clavicul/o)

Scapula (scapul/o)

Sternum (stern/o)

Xiphoid process

Ribs (cost/o)

Thoracic vertebra

Humerus (humer/o)

Lumbar vertebra

Ulna (uln/o)

Ilium (ili/o)

Sacrum (sacr/o)

Coccyx (coccyg/o)

Radius (radi/o)

Carpals (carp/o)

Metacarpals (metacarp/o)

Femur (femor/o)

Phalanges (phalang/o)

Patella (patell/o)

Tibia (tibi/o)

Fibula (fibul/o, perone/o)

Tarsals (tars/o)

Metatarsals (metatars/o)

Calcaneus (calcane/o)

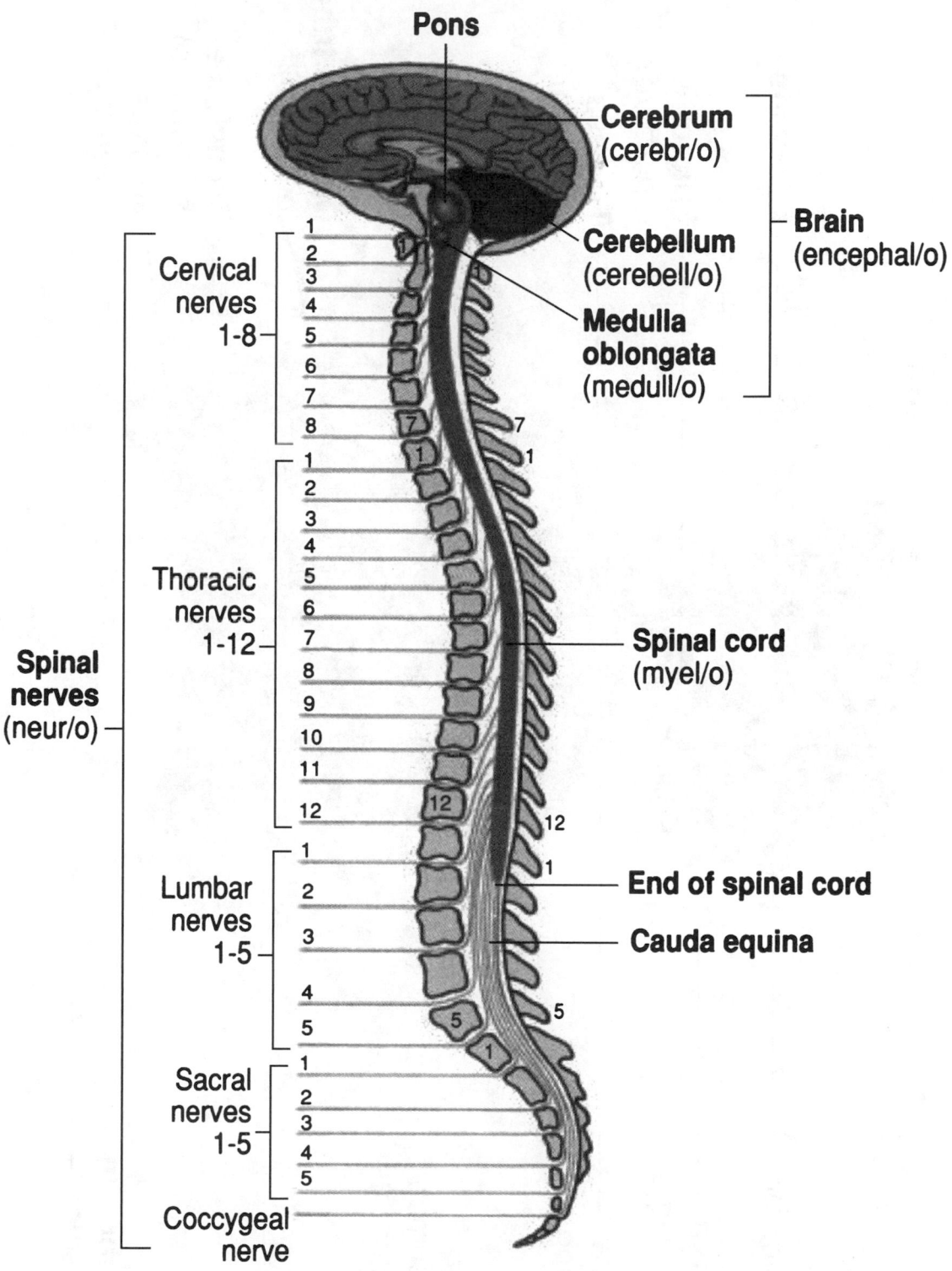

Pons

Cerebrum
(cerebr/o)

Cerebellum
(cerebell/o)

Medulla
oblongata
(medull/o)

Brain
(encephal/o)

Cervical
nerves
1-8

Thoracic
nerves
1-12

Spinal
nerves
(neur/o)

Spinal cord
(myel/o)

Lumbar
nerves
1-5

End of spinal cord

Cauda equina

Sacral
nerves
1-5

Coccygeal
nerve

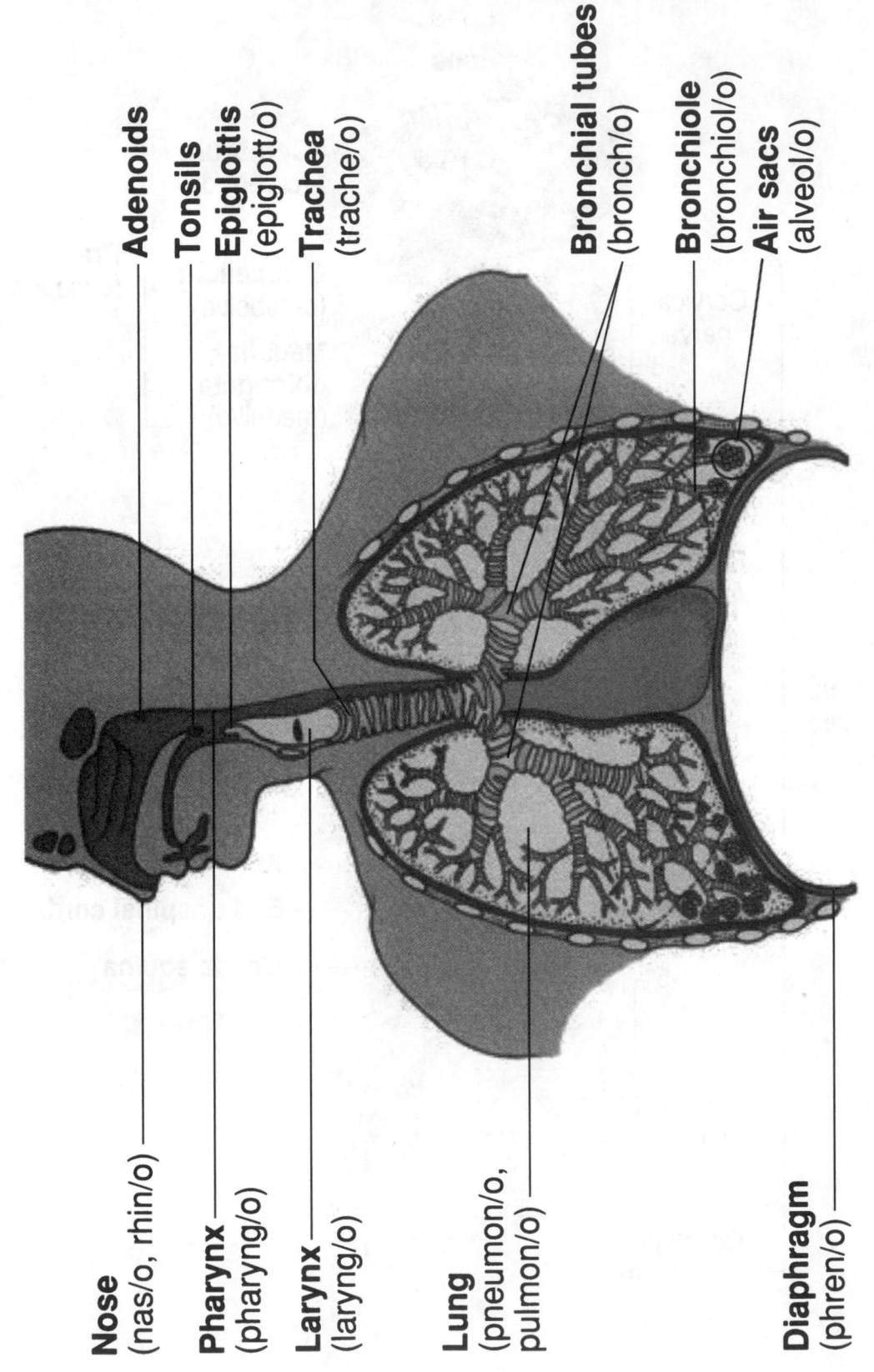

Adenoids

Tonsils

Epiglottis
(epiglott/o)

Trachea
(trache/o)

Bronchial tubes
(bronch/o)

Bronchiole
(bronchiol/o)

Air sacs
(alveol/o)

Nose
(nas/o, rhin/o)

Pharynx
(pharyng/o)

Larynx
(laryng/o)

Lung
(pneumon/o,
pulmon/o)

Diaphragm
(phren/o)

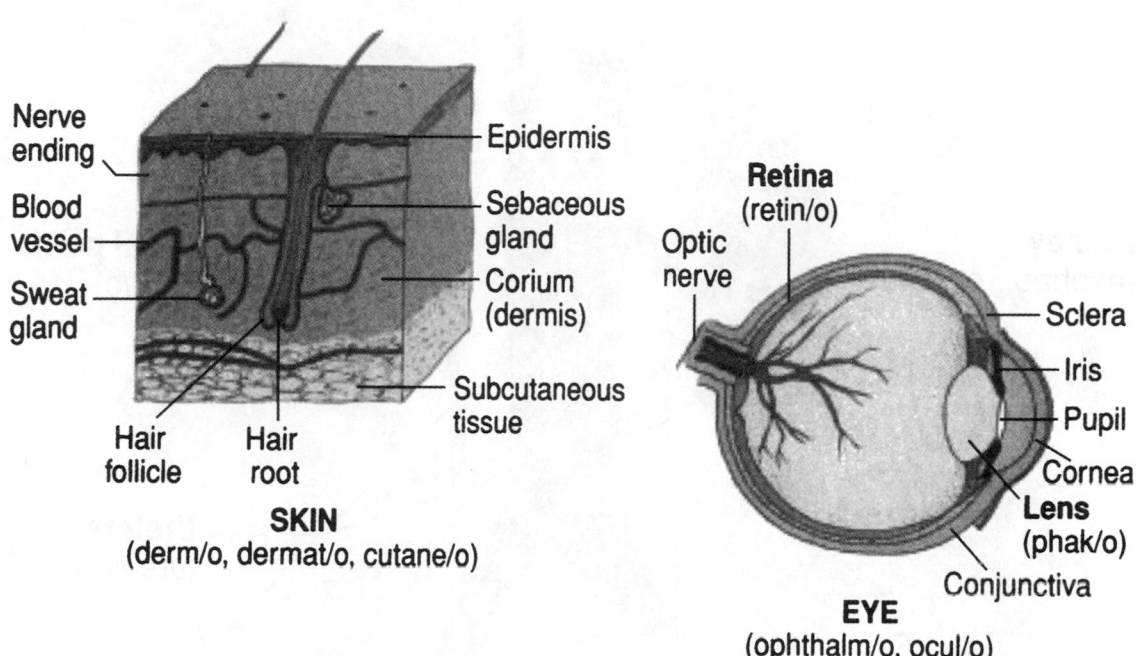

Nerve ending

Blood vessel

Sweat gland

Hair follicle

Hair root

Epidermis

Sebaceous gland

Corium (dermis)

Subcutaneous tissue

SKIN
(derm/o, dermat/o, cutane/o)

Retina
(retin/o)

Optic nerve

Sclera

Iris

Pupil

Cornea

Lens
(phak/o)

Conjunctiva

EYE
(ophthalm/o, ocul/o)

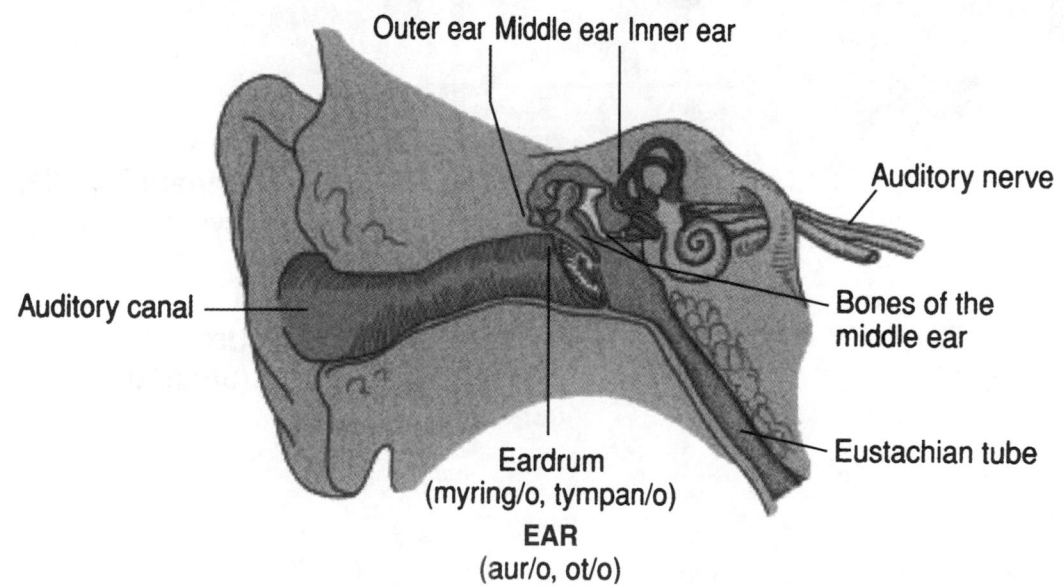

Outer ear   Middle ear   Inner ear

Auditory nerve

Auditory canal

Bones of the middle ear

Eustachian tube

Eardrum
(myring/o, tympan/o)

EAR
(aur/o, ot/o)

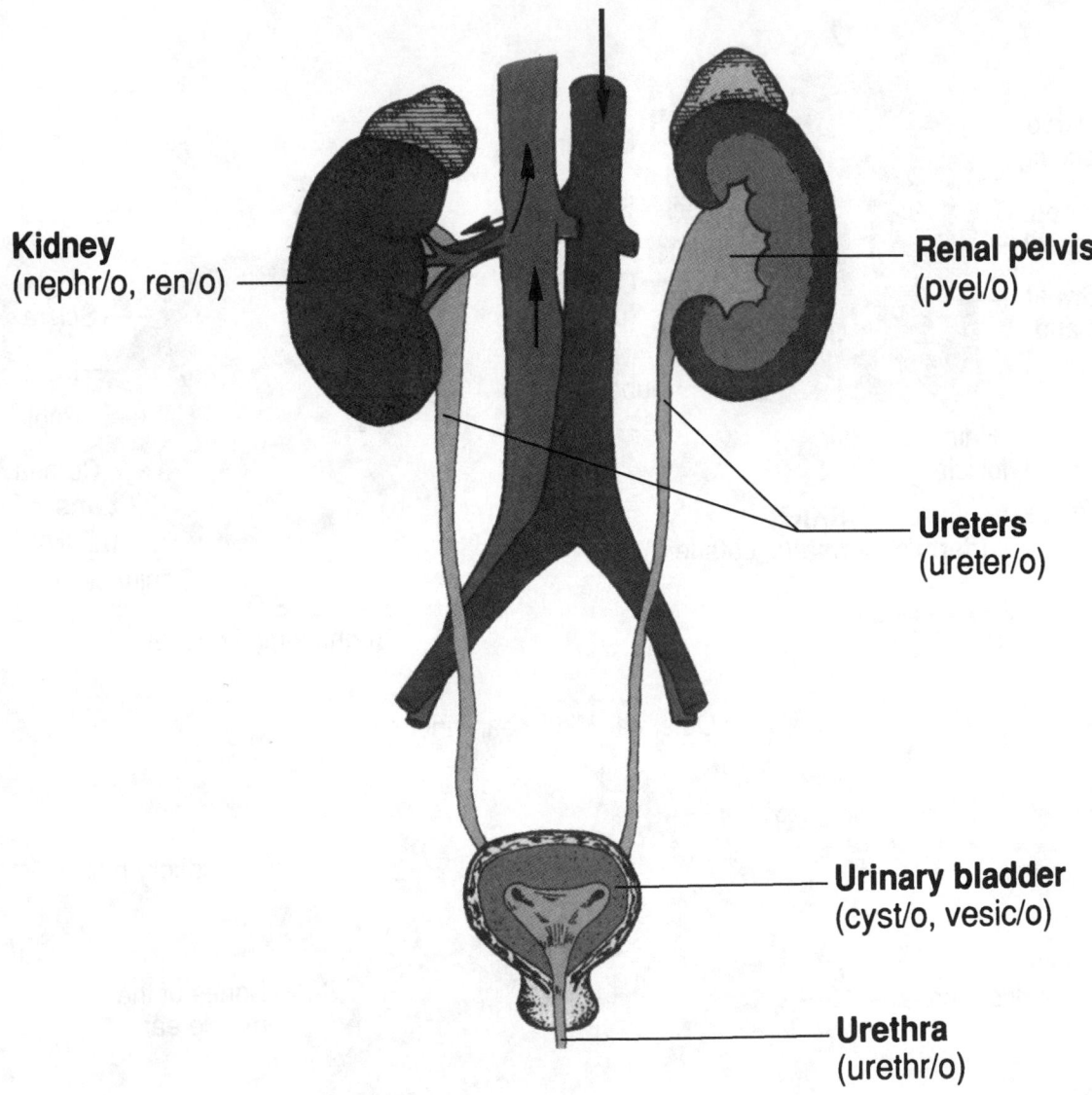

Kidney
(nephr/o, ren/o)

Renal pelvis
(pyel/o)

Ureters
(ureter/o)

Urinary bladder
(cyst/o, vesic/o)

Urethra
(urethr/o)